Medical Complications in Labor and Delivery

In memory of Dad, in honor of Mom, and in appreciation of Cookie, Ilana, Nathan, and Daniel.

B.G.

To my parents and my brother, and especially to Jeff.

R.B.

Medical Complications in Labor and Delivery

Bernard Gonik, MD

Professor and Associate Chairman
Department of Obstetrics and Gynecology
Wayne State University School of
    Medicine
Chief, Department of Obstetrics and
    Gynecology
Grace Hospital/Detroit Medical Center
Detroit, Michigan

Renee A. Bobrowski, MD

Assistant Professor
Division of Maternal-Fetal Medicine
Department of Obstetrics and Gynecology
Wayne State University School of
    Medicine/Hutzel Hospital
Detroit, Michigan

Blackwell
Science

Blackwell Science
Editorial offices:
238 Main Street, Cambridge, Massachusetts 02142, USA
Osney Mead, Oxford OX2 OEL, England
25 John Street, London WC1N 2BL, England
23 Ainslie Place, Edinburgh EH3 6AJ, Scotland
54 University Street, Carlton, Victoria 3053, Australia
Arnette Blackwell SA, 1 rue de Lille, 75007 Paris, France
Blackwell Wissenschafts-Verlag GmbH
Kurfürstendamm 57, 10707 Berlin, Germany
Feldgasse 13, A-1238 Vienna, Austria

Distributors:
North America
Black Science, Inc.
238 Main Street
Cambridge, Massachusetts 02142
(Telephone orders: 800-215-1000 or 617-876-7000)
Australia
Blackwell Science Pty., Ltd.
54 University Street
Carlton, Victoria 3053
(Telephone orders: 03-347-0300)
Outside North America and Australia
Blackwell Science, Ltd.
c/o Marston Book Services, Ltd.
P.O. Box 87
Oxford OX2 0DT
England
(Telephone orders: 44-1865-791155)

Acquisitions: Victoria Reeders
Development: Coleen Traynor
Production: Michelle Choate
Manufacturing: Kathleen Grimes
Typeset by: EPS Group,
Hanover, MD

Printed and bound by Braun-Brumfield, Inc., Ann Arbor, MI

© **1996 by Blackwell Science, Inc.**
Printed in the United States of America
96 97 98 99 5 4 3 2 1

Library of Congress Cataloging-in-Publication Data
Gonik, Bernard.
  Medical complications in labor and delivery / Bernard Gonik, Renee A. Bobrowski.
    p. cm.
  Includes bibliographical references and index.
  ISBN 0-86542-475-6 (pbk.)
    1. Labor (Obstetrics)—Complications. 2. Pregnancy—Complications. 3. Delivery (Obstetrics)—Complications. I. Bobrowski, Renee A. II. Title.
    [DLNM: 1. Labor Complications. 2. Delivery. 3. Pregnancy Complications. WQ 330 G638m 1996]
  RG701.G66 1996
  618.5—dc20
  DNLM/DLC
  for Library of Congress   95-21120
                                                                            CIP

Contents

▼   ▼   ▼   ▼   ▼

Preface

▼   ▼   ▼   ▼   ▼

Any of a variety of medical conditions can complicate the intrapartum period. These conditions can present acutely in labor in the otherwise healthy gravida. On the other hand, many medical complications will have been identified prior to the onset of labor and will necessitate continued care throughout the intrapartum and postpartum periods. Some conditions, by their natural history, will actually mandate induction of labor, and therefore require special attention during the induction and delivery process to minimize maternal and fetal morbidity and mortality. As a general rule, early recognition and control of any medical condition in pregnancy, prior to the onset of labor, will reduce the intrapartum risk to the mother and her fetus. Specific events (i.e., fluid and carbohydrate administration, acute blood loss, stress, bacterial seeding, polypharmacology, etc.) that commonly occur during labor and delivery may adversely affect an otherwise stable medical condition.

This text addresses some of the more common medical complications associated with pregnancy, and is unique in that it focuses on management issues pertaining to the intrapartum period. It is intended to be comprehensive, yet concise and "user friendly." Detailed dialogue on pathophysiology gives way to practical discussions on specific interventional strategies. Throughout the text an attempt was made to present information in table format to improve accessibility. Complete references are supplied at the end of each chapter so that further inquiries can be easily undertaken.

Given the dynamics of obstetrical practice—and the changing medical environment in general—the authors have attempted to present the most current information available. We recognize that opinions vary, individual patient needs must be factored into every management decision, and that new data are always surfacing. It is, therefore, imperative that clinicians take advantage of additional resources in developing management plans for the complicated parturient. We acknowledge the valued input from our many mentors and colleagues who have assisted us in the preparation of this book. The authors welcome correspondence from interested readers, so that future endeavors adequately reflect the broad range of knowledge and expertise available in the scientific and clinical communities.

Bernard Gonik
Renee A. Bobrowski

Hypertensive Disease

▼   ▼   ▼   ▼   ▼

■ PREECLAMPSIA

Pregnancy can induce hypertension in the otherwise normotensive woman, or can aggravate preexisting chronic hypertension. Preeclampsia affects approximately 5% of all pregnancies, and is usually diagnosed by the findings of hypertension in combination with proteinuria or edema (Table 1.1). It is a disease that affects multiple organ systems, including cardiovascular, renal, hematologic, hepatic, and neurologic. The fetus can also be compromised, indirectly via alterations in maternal homeostasis or directly through placental vascular aberrations. At term, in particular with a favorable cervical examination, most authorities would advocate induction of labor since this is the only means by which to resolve this pregnancy complication.

Criteria that classify preeclampsia as severe are listed in Table 1.2. Traditional teachings recommend initiation of labor, regardless of gestational age, when severe preeclampsia is diagnosed. Recent clinical experience, however, suggests favorable maternal and neonatal outcomes after conservative management of carefully selected patients with severe preeclampsia remote from term (1). In these studies, subjects who only had blood pressure abnormalities or proteinuria meeting

Table 1.1 *Criteria for diagnosis of preeclampsia*

Hypertension

Blood pressure ≥ 140/90 mm Hg, taken at least 6 hr apart, after 20 wks gestation *or*

A rise in diastolic pressure ≥ 15 mm Hg *or*

A rise in systolic pressure ≥ 30 mm Hg over baseline blood pressures

Proteinuria

≥ 300 mg/L urinary protein/24 hr *or*

≥ 100 mg/dL in two random urine samples obtained at least 6 hr apart *or*

1–2 ⊕ or greater on qualitative examination

Edema

Clinically evident swelling *or*

Rapid increase in weight (≥ 5 lb/1 wk)

the American College of Obstetricians and Gynecologists' criteria for severe disease were given antihypertensive therapy and intensively monitored in a tertiary perinatal center through 34 weeks' gestation. Guidelines for conservative management based on these data are outlined in Table 1.3.

Initial Evaluation

The intrapartum management of the preeclamptic patient has the following goals: 1) prevention of eclamptic seizures, 2) identification and treatment of associated complications, 3) maintenance of fetal well-being, and 4) delivery of the baby within a reasonable time frame. The

Table 1.2 *Criteria for the diagnosis of severe preeclampsia*

Blood pressure

  ≥ 160 mm Hg systolic *or*

  ≥ 110 mm Hg diastolic

    (recorded on at least two occasions at least 6 hr apart,

    with the patient at bed rest)

Proteinuria

  ≥ 5 gm in 24 hr, *or*

  3–4 ⊕ on qualitative examination

HELLP syndrome

  Hemolysis (abnormal peripheral blood smear, elevated

    bilirubin or increased lactic dehydrogenase)

  Elevated AST or ALT

  Platelet count < 100,000/μL

Oliguria

Cerebral or visual disturbances

Epigastric pain

Pulmonary edema or cyanosis

initial evaluation of a patient with suspected preeclampsia is outlined in Table 1.4. In patients requiring delivery, antiseizure prophylaxis must be instituted without delay and, if necessary, prior to the availability of laboratory results.

The interval at which blood studies are repeated depends on the initial laboratory results and clinical severity of disease. When the results of initial laboratory studies are normal, it is common to repeat these studies

Table 1.3 *Empiric guidelines for conservative management versus immediate delivery in patients with severe preeclampsia remote from term*

Conservative management	Immediate delivery
Maternal parameters	
Controlled hypertension (≤ 160/110 mm Hg)	Uncontrolled hypertension despite adequate therapy
Oliguria responsive to replacement therapy	Thrombocytopenia (platelet count < 100,000/μL)
Mild elevation of AST or ALT without epigastric or right-upper-quadrant pain	Pulmonary edema
	Persistent oliguria or rising serum creatinine level
	Persistent severe headache or visual disturbances
Fetal Parameters	
Biophysical profile ≥ 6	Concerns for fetal well-being
Amniotic fluid index > 2 cm	Oligohydramnios (amniotic fluid index ≤ 2 cm)
Estimated fetal weight > 5th percentile	Suspected severe intrauterine growth restriction
	Reverse umbilical artery diastolic flow

Table 1.4 *Initial evaluation of the patient with suspected preeclampsia*

Assess

Vital signs

Fluid intake and output

Neurologic status

Fetal well-being (nonstress test, amniotic fluid index, and/ or biophysical profile)

Consider

Indwelling bladder catheter

(required in the patient with decreased urine output)

Initial laboratory studies

Hematocrit

Platelet count

Fibrinogen

ALT/AST

Blood type and screen (or crossmatch)

Additional studies as indicated:

Peripheral blood smear

Serum BUN and creatinine

Uric acid

Bilirubin

24-hr urine collection for total protein and creatinine clearance

(for expectantly managed patients)

every 8 to 12 hours, although the clinical utility of this approach is debatable. If the initial studies demonstrate significant abnormalities, it is reasonable to follow these parameters serially throughout the intrapartum and postpartum periods. Vital signs, fluid intake and urine output, and neurologic status should be monitored hourly during labor.

Fluid Management

Fluid management is a central feature in the intrapartum care of the preeclamptic patient. This relates to the underlying pathophysiology of the disease, which can lead to significant vasoconstriction, renal dysfunction, and variable responses to fluid therapy. Clinically, a heterogeneous population of patients in whom intravenous fluids should be used judiciously to prevent iatrogenic injury should be anticipated (2). Ideally, intravenous fluids should be used to replace measurable and insensible losses, and to anticipate intravascular volume depletion due to hemorrhage. Provided that urine output is adequate, it is desirable to maintain the patient in a slightly hypovolemic state. Generally, total fluid requirements will not exceed 125 to 150 mL/hour. The effect of crystalloid and colloid solutions was examined in healthy parturients at term, and there was no apparent clinical benefit to using colloid solution (3). Although preeclampsia is associated with an overall reduction in colloid osmotic pressure, it is unlikely that under these circumstances the choice of intravenous solution is of clinical importance.

The presence of oliguria may complicate fluid management in the preeclamptic patient. Unfortunately, urinary diagnostic indices such as specific gravity and fractional excretion of sodium are poor predictors of intravascular volume status in these patients (4). Therefore, fluid management under these conditions may require central hemodynamic monitoring, as discussed later.

Seizure Prophylaxis

In 1906, magnesium sulfate was first reported as an intrathecal injection for the prevention of eclampsia. Currently, it remains the drug of choice in North America for the prevention and treatment of seizures associated with preeclampsia. Opponents of its use believe that magnesium has no central inhibition of seizure foci but acts only via peripheral neuromuscular blockade. However, Cotton et al (5) recently demonstrated the central anticonvulsant activity of magnesium sulfate in an animal model via suppression of the N-methyl-D-aspartate receptor of the hippocampus. Phenytoin as well as other anticonvulsants and sedatives have been suggested as alternative therapies (6). Sibai (7) reviewed the controversy over the ideal anticonvulsant, and provided evidence for the safety, efficacy, and familiarity of magnesium sulfate. Since 20% of eclamptic women may have minimal blood pressure elevations and no proteinuria, all women diagnosed with preeclampsia should receive antiseizure prophylaxis during labor. The American College of Obstetricians and Gynecologists considers seizure prophylaxis with magnesium sulfate to be the standard of care in the management of preeclampsia (8).

Magnesium sulfate is most commonly administered as an intravenous solution. Protocols for intramuscular injection of magnesium were utilized previously, but are no longer preferred in institutions where adequate monitoring is available. Intravenous magnesium solutions should be administered via an infusion pump to prevent accidental toxicity. A loading dose of 4 to 6 gm over 20 minutes followed by a maintenance dose of 2 gm/hour is advocated by Sibai (7). Although there are no definite guidelines, magnesium is generally continued for 24 to 48 hours following delivery to prevent postpartum eclampsia. Anecdotal experiences suggest that magnesium sulfate can be safely discontinued earlier in the postpartum period when a patient with nonsevere preeclampsia demonstrates evidence of resolving symptomatology.

Therapeutic serum levels of magnesium range from 4 to 7 mg/dL, although the clinical utility of routine measurement of these levels is unclear. Conversely, since magnesium excretion is almost exclusively renal, patients with decreased urine output must be monitored more closely with scheduled measurements. The magnesium infusion should be stopped and serum levels of magnesium obtained if clinical signs of toxicity are noted. Toxicity will become clinically apparent when serum magnesium levels reach 9 to 12 mg/dL and deep tendon reflexes are lost. Other symptoms may include nausea, somnolence, double vision, and slurred speech. Respiratory depression and cardiac arrest occur at magnesium levels above 15 and 30 mg/dL, respectively. Treatment of magnesium toxicity includes: 1) respiratory support with oxygen or endotracheal intubation and mechanical ventilation when clinically indicated, 2) infusion of calcium salts (10 mL of a 10% calcium gluconate solution), 3) continuous cardiac monitoring, and

4) administration of a loop or osmotic diuretic to increase magnesium excretion (9).

Antihypertensive Therapy

The main objective in treating preeclampsia-associated hypertension is prevention of cerebral hemorrhage, cardiac decompensation, and abruptio placentae. Acute medical therapy (Table 1.5) should be instituted for diastolic blood pressures above 110 mm Hg; many authorities recommend treatment when systolic pressures are above 170 to 180 mm Hg. The goal is to reduce and maintain diastolic pressure in the range of 90 to 105 mm Hg; this is presumed to minimize the risk of compromising uteroplacental perfusion. Although magnesium sulfate is a mainstay in the treatment of preeclampsia, it is not an effective antihypertensive agent. A bolus of magnesium has been shown to have a transient hypotensive effect on mean arterial pressure, but this effect is lost by 1 hour even with continued infusion (10).

Hydralazine hydrochloride (Apresoline) is the antihypertensive agent with the most extensive clinical experience in pregnancy. It is a direct vasodilator of arteriolar smooth muscle. The initial intravenous dose of 5 mg should be allowed 20 minutes for the full hemodynamic effect. When severe hypertension persists, an additional 5- to 10-mg bolus can be given at 20-minute intervals until blood pressure is controlled or a total of 40 mg has been administered. A dosing interval closer than 20 minutes may result in significant hypotension. Alternatively, a continuous infusion starting at 1 mg/hour can be used for blood pressure control. Adverse reactions include tachycardia, palpitations, nausea, and headache.

Table 1.5 *Acute antihypertensive therapy*

Drug	Action	Dose	Maximum dose	Adverse reaction	Time to effect
Hydralazine	Direct vasodilator	Initial: 5 mg IVP Repeat: 5–10 mg q20min	40 mg	Tachycardia, nausea, headache	20 min
Labetalol	Alpha-1 and beta blockade	Initial: 20 mg IVP Repeat: 40–80 mg q10min	300 mg	Postural hypotension	10 min
Nifedipine	Calcium channel blocker	Initial: 10 mg SL Repeat: 10 mg SL 30 min after initial dose	180 mg/day	Hypotension when given with $MgSO_4$	10–20 min
Nitroglycerin	Venous dilator at low dose Arterial dilator at high dose	Initial: 5 μg/min, continuous infusion Increase: Double dose q3–5 min	Undetermined	Methemoglobinemia at > 7 μg/kg/min	3–5 min
Nitroprusside	Venodilator	Initial: 0.25 μg/kg/min Increase 0.25 μg/kg/min q5 min	10 μg/kg/min	Cyanide toxicity, methemoglobinemia	1–5 min

IVP = intravenous push; SL = sublingually.

Hydralazine is contraindicated in women with coronary artery disease because it may result in reflex tachycardia. Although hydralazine will adequately control hypertension in most patients, second-line therapy is indicated when blood pressures are refractory to maximal doses.

Labetalol hydrochloride (Trandate, Normodyne) produces a combined alpha-1 and beta-receptor blockade. Both oral and intravenous administration result in a more potent beta- than alpha-1 blockade effect. Studies have documented the efficacy and safety of labetalol for the treatment of hypertension in pregnancy (11–13). Mabie (11) demonstrated the effectiveness of labetalol in managing severe hypertension associated with preeclampsia. Labetalol has several advantages when compared to hydralazine, including a more rapid onset of action when administered intravenously and less reflex tachycardia and maternal hypotension. No alterations in uteroplacental perfusion have been observed (14). The initial dose of labetalol is 20 mg intravenously, with a maximal effect usually noted by 20 minutes. If, after the initial injection, no response is noted in 10 minutes, doses can be increased from 40 to 80 mg until blood pressure control is achieved or a maximum dose of 300 mg is given. Considerable interpatient variation has been reported in dosing requirements, and was not predictable by any specific clinical characteristic (11). Labetalol can also be administered as a continuous infusion at a rate of 1 to 2 mg/min, titrated to the desired blood pressure range.

The calcium channel blocker nifedipine (Procardia) reduces blood pressure by blocking the slow calcium channel and relaxing smooth muscle. Sublingual nifedipine (10 mg) can be administered for the initial management of severe hypertension. Blood pressure reduction occurs in 10 to 20 minutes. A second sublingual dose of 10 mg may be administered 30 minutes after the initial dose, if needed. Due to the risk of severe hypotension, nifedipine must be administered with caution to a patient receiving magnesium sulfate (15). The use of nifedipine in the intrapartum period has not been tested in a controlled clinical trial. Barton et al (16), however, reported on the use of nifedipine during the postpartum period for patients with severe preeclampsia. They noted that mean arterial pressure decreased and urine output increased significantly in treated versus control patients when nifedipine was begun in the immediate postpartum period.

Nitroglycerin and sodium nitroprusside are two additional second-line antihypertensive agents that are particularly useful for treating hypertensive crises or controlling severe hypertension associated with tracheal intubation. Since these two agents have a rapid onset of action and short hemodynamic half-lives, monitoring with an arterial line to assist in the titration of these drugs is usually performed. Nitroglycerin is a venous dilator at doses of 30 to 40 μg/minute and an arteriolar dilator at higher doses (> 250 μg/min). The infusion of nitroglycerin should begin at 5 μg/minute; the dose can be doubled every 3 to 5 minutes. A limited number of studies on the use of this agent for preeclampsia have been conducted. In severe preeclamptic patients, Cotton et al (17) noted that the dosage requirement of nitroglycerin for blood pressure reduction was inversely related to the patient's volume status. Volume expansion in combination with nitroglycerin allowed for the maintenance of cardiac index, pulmonary wedge pressure, and oxygen utilization. Nitroglycerin may be associated with a precipitous reduction in blood pressure and the development of methemoglobinemia at doses higher than 7 μg/kg/minute. An arterial methemoglobin level should be determined in any patient with cyanosis and normal arterial oxygen saturation. Toxic levels above 3% should be treated with 1 to 2 mg of intravenous methylene blue per kilogram.

Sodium nitroprusside is administered at an initial dose of 0.25 μg/kg/minute and increased 0.25 μg/kg/minute every 5 minutes to a maximum of 10 μg/kg/minute. Prior to administration of nitroprusside, hypovolemia must be corrected to avoid profound hypotension. Complications of nitroprusside include cyanide toxicity and methemoglobinemia; the risk of either complication can be avoided with short-term administration. A patient with cyanide toxicity may experience air hunger and appear confused. Arterial blood gases should be monitored for metabolic acidosis, which is an early sign of toxicity. Venous hyperoxia (bright red venous blood) is due to decreased cellular extraction of oxygen. Evaluation of a patient with signs and symptoms of cyanide toxicity includes arterial blood gas analysis and determination of plasma cyanide, red cell cyanide, and methemoglobin levels. Due to the potential for both maternal and fetal toxicity, nitroprusside should be used only when other antihypertensive agents have failed to control blood pressure.

Hematologic Abnormalities

A variety of isolated and combined hematologic abnormalities have been associated with preeclampsia. Most of these are important only in that they define the severity of the condition, and do not require specific therapy as spontaneous resolution is anticipated after delivery. It is important to recognize HELLP (hemolysis, elevated liver enzymes, and low platelets) syndrome and differentiate it from other disease processes that can mimic this syndrome (Table 1.6). Laboratory abnormalities can occur in the absence of overt hypertension; 20% of patients demonstrating HELLP syndrome have normal blood pressure and 30% have only mild blood pressure elevation (18). Thirty-one percent of patients do not develop HELLP until the postpartum period and represent a group at increased risk for developing pulmonary edema and acute renal failure. The syndrome has also been associated with increased maternal and fetal morbidity and mortality.

Thrombocytopenia (platelet count < 100,000/mm) (3) occurs in 9.7 to 16.0% of patients with preeclampsia (19–21). The incidence approaches 30% in patients with eclampsia (22). Patients with thrombocytopenia are at greatest risk for coagulation abnormalities and warrant assessment of prothrombin time (PT), partial thromboplastin time (PTT), and fibrinogen. Leduc et al (23) noted that patients whose platelet count was higher than 100,000/mm (3) had a low risk for coagulopathy and therefore did not require further screening. In patients with thrombocytopenia, Neiger et al (24) reported that mean nadir levels were reached 27 hours following delivery. Recovery time appeared to be inversely related to the level of the thrombocytopenia, with the mean time of 60 hours required for platelet counts to return to more than 100,000/mm (3).

Table 1.6 *Differential diagnosis of HELLP syndrome*

	Leukocytosis	Thrombo-cytopenia	Elevated liver enzyme levels	Hemolysis	Jaundice	Disseminated intravascular coagulation	Disease-specific findings
HELLP	−	++	+	++	−	+/−	Associated with preeclampsia
Acute fatty liver of pregnancy	+++	+/−	++	−	++	++	Hypoglycemia, elevated ammonia
Hepatitis	++	−	+++	−	+++	+/−	Large, tender liver
Abruption	+/−	+	−	−	−	++	Vaginal bleeding, fetal distress
Hemolytic-uremic syndrome	+	+++	−	++	+	−	Significant renal dysfunction
Thrombotic thrombocytopenic purpura	++	+++	−	++	+	−	Neurologic aberrations

Platelet transfusion is indicated for any patient with a platelet count lower than 20,000/mm (3) or with active bleeding regardless of platelet count. Patients who undergo cesarean section should have a platelet count of at least 50,000/mm (3). Transfusion of 10 units of platelets should be initiated just prior to the skin incision for any patient with a platelet count lower than 50,000/mm (3). Repeated platelet transfusions are not indicated because of rapid consumption and increased risk for antibody formation. Generalized oozing from the operative site is common, and a subfacial closed-drainage system may be appropriate in some situations. Sibai (18) recommended a delayed skin closure at 72 hours given the 20% incidence of hematoma formation.

Hemolysis results from passage of red blood cells through damaged blood vessels. In HELLP syndrome, the hemolysis usually does not result in anemia requiring blood transfusion. Elevated liver transaminase levels are found in 21 to 31% of preeclamptic patients (25). The alkaline phosphatase level is normally elevated during pregnancy and thus offers little additional clinical information. Since alanine aminotransferase (ALT) and aspartate aminotransferase (AST) rise in parallel with HELLP syndrome, consideration can be given to serial measurements of one of these two parameters.

The principal management of patients with HELLP syndrome is supportive in nature. Blood component therapy is not usually based on any absolute laboratory value. Fresh frozen plasma and cryoprecipitate, however, are traditionally utilized to maintain the fibrinogen level above 100 mg/dL. Platelet replacement therapy should be carried out according to the previously suggested guidelines. The presence of HELLP syndrome alone is not an indication for cesarean delivery. Patients in spontaneous labor may be delivered vaginally. Induction of labor with oxytocin is appropriate, although given the progression of this disease, some arbitrary time limitation should be established for the initiation of active labor and delivery. These parameters must be individualized to the condition of the patient and the fetus.

Oliguria

Transient renal dysfunction is common in patients with preeclampsia, but fortunately, permanent renal injury is an uncommon event. Renal abnormalities may result from hypovolemia, renal artery vasospasm, renal injury, or their combination. Oliguria is the most frequent clinical indicator suggesting compromise of this organ system. Although the standard definition of oliguria is a urine output of less than 400 mL/24 hours, for intrapartum management considerations, it is often defined as urine output of less than 30 mL/hour for 2 consecutive hours.

The initial management of oliguria should take into consideration whether this finding requires intervention. Absolute criteria have not been established for pregnancy, but clinical experience suggests that preeclamptic patients can tolerate this condition for a short period of time without the risk of permanent injury. Therefore, if delivery is imminent, treatment of oliguria can be delayed until the postpartum period, in anticipation of spontaneous resolution.

If the patient is remote from delivery or it is essential

to know the intravascular volume status (e.g., prior to conduction anesthesia), a more aggressive approach must be undertaken in the oliguric patient. A careful fluid challenge of 500 to 1000 mL of crystalloid solution can be administered over 20 to 30 minutes. As previously discussed, urinary diagnostic indices (urine osmolality, sodium, specific gravity, urine/plasma creatinine and urea nitrogen, and fractional excretion of sodium) have not proved useful in determining volume status in preeclamptic women. Therefore, if urine output has not responded to the initial empiric 1000-mL fluid challenge, pulmonary artery catheterization is indicated for the further assessment of intravascular volume status. Repetitive fluid challenges without invasive monitoring can result in rapid development of pulmonary edema.

Through invasive hemodynamic monitoring, three subsets of patients with preeclampsia complicated by oliguria have been described (2). Patients in group I had low to low-normal pulmonary capillary wedge pressure (PCWP), hyperdynamic left ventricular function, and moderately elevated systemic vascular resistance (SVR). Oliguria appeared to be based on relative intravascular volume depletion with systemic arteriospasm; these patients responded to a fluid challenge. It was believed that this group represents the majority of oliguric preeclamptic women who respond to a fluid bolus without requiring invasive monitoring. Group II included patients with a high-normal to elevated PCWP and normal SVR; this suggests selective renal arteriospasm, which does not respond to volume expansion. Afterload reduction with hydralazine and careful fluid administration resulted in increased urine output. The third group had an elevated PCWP, depressed left ventricular function, and elevated SVR, which required fluid restriction and afterload reduction for correction of oliguria. Kirshon et al (26) demonstrated that low-dose dopamine increases urine output in this last group of patients, and thus may be of benefit in resolving the oliguria.

Pulmonary Edema

Pulmonary edema is diagnosed on the basis of signs of respiratory distress, pulmonary rales, hypoxemia as defined by a partial arterial oxygen pressure lower than 70 mm Hg on room air, and radiographic changes. It has been reported to occur in 2.9% of patients with severe preeclampsia/eclampsia and is associated with high maternal and perinatal morbidity and mortality (27). Pulmonary edema often presents during the postpartum period. It occurs more frequently in older and multigravid women, patients with chronic hypertension, and following excessive intravenous fluid administration. Invasive hemodynamic monitoring has demonstrated that the most common reason for pulmonary edema in preeclampsia is a lowered colloid oncotic pressure (COP)–PCWP gradient (28), with a COP–PCWP gradient of 4 mm Hg or less increasing the likelihood (29).

The initial management of pulmonary edema includes oxygen administration, continuous pulse oximetry, placement of a urinary catheter, careful monitoring of intake and output, fluid restriction, and diuresis. Early treatment of pulmonary edema is important. Aside from the resultant hypoxia, prolonged capillary leakage can lead to development of adult respiratory distress syndrome. The initial dose of furosemide (Lasix) is 10 to

40 mg over 2 minutes. If adequate diuresis does not follow within 1 hour, the initial dose may be doubled. In
the event of aggressive diuresis, serum electrolyte levels
should be serially monitored. When hypoxemia persists
despite initial therapy, mechanical ventilation is required. An arterial line may assist with serial blood gas
monitoring, and a pulmonary artery catheter will facilitate determination of the underlying pathophysiologic
mechanism responsible for the pulmonary edema.
Although not all patients with pulmonary edema require
invasive monitoring, it should be strongly considered in
a patient who does not respond to initial therapy.

Central Nervous System Complications

Cerebral edema occurs secondary to increased intravascular pressure, decreased COP, damaged vascular endo-
thelium, or a combination of these factors. The edema
associated with preeclampsia may be due to the loss of
cerebral autoregulation secondary to severe hypertension or anoxia associated with eclamptic seizures (30).
Low COP found with eclampsia may be a contributing
factor in the diffuse cerebral edema seen following
seizures.

The treatment of cerebral edema consists of correction of hypoxia and hypercarbia, control of blood pressure and body temperature, and avoidance of volatile
anesthetics. Mechanical hyperventilation to maintain a
partial carbon dioxide pressure of 25 to 30 mm Hg
reduces cerebral edema. Osmotic agents such as mannitol reduce intracranial water and volume by a fluid
shift from the extravascular to the intravascular compartment. Mannitol is administered intravenously at a

dose of 0.5 to 1.0 gm/kg of body weight over 10 minutes. Alternatively, it can be given as a continuous intravenous infusion of 5 gm/hour. Serum osmolality should be maintained between 305 and 315 mOsm. Steroid therapy is less beneficial in patients with acute diffuse cerebral edema of preeclampsia than in those with chronic focal edema seen with a tumor or abscess. Thus, steroids are not recommended in the preeclamptic patient with cerebral edema (31).

Cerebral hemorrhage resulting from severe hypertension is associated with a high mortality rate. Control of seizure activity and hypertension, and ventilatory support should occur in an intensive care setting. Laboratory studies to detect disseminated intravascular coagulopathy (DIC) should be performed, as this will only worsen the hemorrhagic condition. Although acute surgical intervention is rarely beneficial, neurosurgical consultation should be obtained.

Anesthesia in Patients with Preeclampsia

Intravenous analgesics are commonly used in patients with preeclampsia for pain relief during labor. Narcotics are often administered in combination with phenothiazines, but the latter must be used cautiously because of the theoretical lowering of the seizure threshold.

The use of epidural anesthesia has been questioned on the basis that sympathetic blockade combined with intravascular volume contraction will cause maternal hypotension and resultant poor placental perfusion. Jouppila et al (32), however, demonstrated that intervillous blood flow significantly improved following epidural analgesia. Doppler studies of the umbilical artery suggested that epidural anesthesia in preeclamptic patients is associated with a reduction in placental resistance and may actually benefit the fetus (33). Cautious use of epidural anesthesia for labor and nonemergent cesarean section is supported by both anesthesiologists and obstetricians. Placement early in the course of labor can decrease the need for emergent induction of general anesthesia with its associated risks. Prior to catheter placement, the patient should be in the left lateral position and have received 500 to 1500 mL of intravenous crystalloid. Fetal monitoring should be continuous during establishment of anesthesia to detect selective uterine hypotension and fetal distress. Ephedrine is the treatment of choice for maternal hypotension. Anesthetic levels should be segmentally achieved to decrease the risk of hypotension. Contraindications to epidural anesthesia include: 1) thrombocytopenia or coagulopathy, 2) systemic infection, 3) fetal distress, or 4) patient request for alternative method of pain relief.

General endotracheal anesthesia produces a significant rise in systemic arterial blood pressure and PCWP with severe preeclampsia (34). In addition to the usual risks of general anesthesia in pregnancy, severe hypertension in response to laryngoscopy, laryngeal edema, and the interaction of magnesium sulfate with anesthetic agents increase the risk of complications.

Invasive Monitoring

Patients with severe preeclampsia or eclampsia complicated by unexplained oliguria, pulmonary edema, or refractory hypertension requiring nitroprusside or nitroglycerin are candidates for invasive hemodynamic monitoring. When volume status is uncertain, placement of a pulmonary artery catheter is recommended given the poor correlation between central venous pressure and pulmonary capillary wedge pressure (35–36). Although this catheter has never been tested in a randomized controlled trial, it does enable the clinician to assess more accurately a patient's volume status and determine the underlying pathophysiology of the pulmonary edema or oliguria.

The typical patient with severe preeclampsia has a high SVR and cardiac output. This high output is secondary to increased heart rate and stroke volume. However, patients with severe preeclampsia demonstrate a continuum from high-output low-resistance to low-output high-resistance states (35–39). This variation appears to be independent of the effects of intravenous magnesium sulfate therapy, but may represent other pharmacologic interventions prior to invasive monitoring. Table 1.7 outlines the typical hemodynamic profile of a patient with severe preeclampsia.

Invasive monitoring can aid in differentiating cardiogenic and noncardiogenic pulmonary edema. Cardiogenic pulmonary edema can result from iatrogenic fluid overload or left ventricular failure associated with very high SVR. Pulmonary edema caused by fluid overload will benefit from diuresis, whereas severe systemic vasospasm will respond optimally to afterload reduction. Noncardiogenic pulmonary edema is best treated by lowering the PCWP to the lowest level that will continue to maintain adequate cardiac output.

ECLAMPSIA

Standard therapy for a patient with eclampsia includes seizure and blood pressure control, and plans to deliver

Table 1.7 *Hemodynamic parameters in patients with preeclampsia*

Hemodynamic Parameter	Normal pregnancy*	Change from normal pregnancy
Cardiac output	6.2 ± 1.0 L/min	Variable
Mean arterial pressure	90.3 ± 5.8 mm Hg	Increased
Central venous pressure	3.6 ± 2.5 mm Hg	Low to normal
Pulmonary capillary wedge pressure	7.5 ± 1.8 mm Hg	Variable
Systemic vascular resistance	1210 ± 266 dyne × cm × sec^{-5}	Normal to elevated
Left ventricular stroke work index	41 ± 8 gm × m × m^{-2}	Usually increased
Colloid oncotic pressure	18.0 ± 1.5 mm Hg	Decreased

* Modified from Clark SL, Cotton DB, Lee W, et al. Central hemodynamic assessment of normal term pregnancy. Am J Obstet Gynecol 1989; 161:1439.

the fetus (Table 1.8). Magnesium sulfate is given as a 4- to 6-gm intravenous loading dose followed by a maintenance infusion of 2 gm/hour. Should a patient have a convulsion after receiving this initial dose, a second bolus of 2 to 4 gm may be administered over 5 minutes. If convulsions continue after the second magnesium bolus, amobarbital sodium, a short-acting barbiturate,

Table 1.8 *Initial intravenous pharmacologic approach to eclampsia*

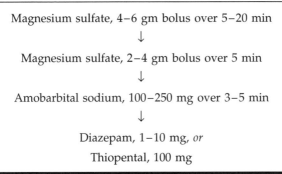

Magnesium sulfate, 4–6 gm bolus over 5–20 min
↓
Magnesium sulfate, 2–4 gm bolus over 5 min
↓
Amobarbital sodium, 100–250 mg over 3–5 min
↓
Diazepam, 1–10 mg, *or*
Thiopental, 100 mg

should be given intravenously in a dose up to 250 mg over 3 to 5 minutes. Intravenous thiopental sodium (100 mg) and diazepam (1–10 mg) are alternative therapies for continued convulsions. Diazepam should be used with caution given the increased risk of maternal and neonatal respiratory depression. Indications for obtaining a computed tomography scan of the head in a patient with eclampsia are not clearly defined, but refractory seizures or focal neurologic signs may warrant consideration of diagnostic imaging after the patient is stabilized.

During a seizure, it is important to insert a padded tongue blade, maintain the patient's airway, clear secretions, and administer oxygen. Fetal bradycardia is commonly associated with seizure activity. The bradycardia results from the combined effects of sustained uterine contractions, maternal hypoxia, and uterine artery vasospasm. Fetal heart rate abnormalities have been reported to last up to 9 minutes (40). Although it is tempting to proceed with emergent cesarean section when there is an abnormal fetal heart tracing during a seizure, an adequate recovery period should be allowed. If the fetus continues to show signs of compromise following control of the convulsion and restoration of maternal oxygenation, delivery can be performed.

The current standard in the management of a patient with eclampsia is to initiate delivery after maternal stabilization. This condition does not preclude vaginal delivery. Pritchard et al (29) noted that 67% of patients with eclampsia delivered vaginally, including patients with preterm fetuses and those requiring induction of labor. Unless the maternal condition is rapidly deteriorating, cesarean section should be reserved for standard obstetric indications.

■ CHRONIC HYPERTENSION

Chronic hypertension is one of the most common medical diseases complicating pregnancy. It is associated with an increased risk of superimposed preeclampsia, abruptio placentae, and fetal growth retardation. The overall incidence of superimposed preeclampsia is 20 to 30%, with the highest risk in patients with severe hypertension. The 15% risk of preeclampsia in the gravida with mild to moderate hypertension does not appear to be decreased by antenatal treatment with methyldopa (Aldomet) or labetalol (41). The risk of abruptio is approximately 5% with chronic hypertension but increases to 15% when preeclampsia is also present.

Intrapartum management of the patient with chronic

hypertension is aimed at blood pressure control, early detection of superimposed preeclampsia, and intensive fetal surveillance with continuous fetal monitoring. Patients who have been well controlled during the antenatal period may be continued on their regimen through labor and delivery. Acute fluctuations in maternal blood pressure can be controlled with the intravenous antihypertensive agents, as discussed under preeclampsia. An arterial line may be beneficial when blood pressure is difficult to control and does not respond to initial therapy. Close attention must be given to intravenous fluid administration and urine output. Epidural anesthesia is an acceptable method of pain relief, but hypotension must be avoided to prevent fetal compromise.

Women requiring multiple antihypertensive agents and those with cardiac disease, chronic renal disease, second-trimester superimposed preeclampsia, or abruptio placentae with DIC are at significantly increased risk to develop postpartum complications. This group should be observed closely during the initial 48 hours after delivery for development of hypertensive encephalopathy, pulmonary edema, and renal failure. Severe hypertension should be controlled with intravenous agents as required. Diuretic therapy has been recommended for massively obese women with long-standing hypertension and those with previous postpartum pulmonary edema (42).

REFERENCES

1. Schiff E, Friedman SA, Sibai BM. Conservative management of severe preeclampsia remote from term. Obstet Gynecol 1994;84:626–630.

2. Clark SL, Greenspoon JS, Aldahl D, Phelan JP. Severe preeclampsia with persistent oliguria: management of hemodynamic subsets. Am J Obstet Gynecol 1986;154: 490–494.

3. Jones MM, Longmire S, Cotton DB, Dorman KF, Skjonsby BS, Joyce TH III. Influence of crystalloid versus colloid infusion on peripartum colloid osmotic pressure changes. Obstet Gynecol 1986;86:659–661.

4. Lee W, Gonik B, Cotton DB. Urinary diagnostic indices in preeclampsia-associated oliguria: correlation with invasive hemodynamic monitoring. Am J Obstet Gynecol 1987;156:100–103.

5. Cotton DB, Janusz CA, Berman RF. Anticonvulsant effects of magnesium sulfate on hippocampal seizures: therapeutic implications in preeclampsia-eclampsia. Am J Obstet Gynecol 1992;166:1127–1136.

6. Lewis PJ, Bulpitt CJ, Zuspan FP. A comparison of current British and American practice in the management of hypertension in pregnancy. Br J Obstet Gynaecol 1980;1: 78–82.

7. Sibai BM. Magnesium sulfate is the ideal anticonvulsant in preeclampsia-eclampsia. Am J Obstet Gynecol 1990;162: 1141–1145.

8. Management of preeclampsia. ACOG Technical Bulletin No. 91. American College of Obstetricians and Gynecologists, Washington, D.C., February 1986.

9. Bohman VR, Cotton DB. Supralethal magnesemia with patient survival. Obstet Gynecol 1990;76:984–985.

10. Cotton DB, Gonik B, Dorman KF. Cardiovascular alterations in severe pregnancy-induced hypertension: acute effects of intravenous magnesium sulfate. Am J Obstet Gynecol 1984;148:162–165.

11. Mabie WC, Gonzalez AR, Sibai BM, Amon E. A comparative trial of labetalol and hydralazine in the acute man-

agement of severe hypertension complicating pregnancy. Obstet Gynecol 1987;70:328–333.

12. Plouin PF, Breart G, Maillard F, Papiernik E, Relier JP. Comparison of antihypertensive efficacy and perinatal safety of labetalol and methyldopa in the treatment of hypertension in pregnancy: a randomized controlled trial. Br J Obstet Gynaecol 1988;95:868–876.

13. Pickles CJ, Symonds EM, Broughton Pipkin F. The fetal outcome in a randomized trial of labetalol versus placebo in pregnancy-induced hypertension. Br J Obstet Gynaecol 1989;96:38–43.

14. Lunell NO, Nylund L, Lewander R, Sarby B. Acute effect of an antihypertensive drug, labetalol, on uteroplacental blood flow. Br J Obstet Gynaecol 1982;89:640–644.

15. Waisman GD, Mayorga LM, Camera MI, Vignolo CA, Martinotti A. Magnesium plus nifedipine: potentiation of hypotensive effect in preeclampsia? Am J Obstet Gynecol 1988;159:308–309.

16. Barton JR, Hiett AK, Conover WB. The use of nifedipine during the postpartum period in patients with severe preeclampsia. Am J Obstet Gynecol 1990;162:788–792.

17. Cotton DB, Longmire S, Jones MM, Dorman KF, Tessem J, Joyce TH III. Cardiovascular alterations in severe pregnancy-induced hypertension: effects of intravenous nitroglycerin coupled with blood volume expansion. Am J Obstet Gynecol 1986;154:1053–1059.

18. Sibai BS. The HELLP syndrome (hemolysis, elevated liver enzymes, and low platelets): much ado about nothing? Am J Obstet Gynecol 1990;162:311–316.

19. Romero R, Mazor M, Lockwood CJ, et al. Clinical significance, prevalence, and natural history of thrombocytopenia in pregnancy-induced hypertension. Am J Perinatol 1989;6:32–38.

20. Katz VL, Thorp JM Jr, Rozas L, Bowes WA Jr. The natural

history of thrombocytopenia associated with preeclampsia. Am J Obstet Gynecol 1990;163:1142–1143.

21. Sibai BM, Taslimi MM, El-Nazer A, Amon E, Mabie BC, Ryan GM. Maternal-perinatal outcome associated with the syndrome of hemolysis, elevated liver enzymes, and low platelets in severe preeclampsia-eclampsia. Am J Obstet Gynecol 1986;155:501–509.

22. Pritchard JA, Cunningham FG, Mason RA. Coagulation changes in eclampsia: their frequency and pathogenesis. Am J Obstet Gynecol 1976:124:855–864.

23. Leduc L, Wheeler JM, Kirshon B, Mitchell P, Cotton DB. Coagulation profile in severe preeclampsia. Obstet Gynecol 1992;79:14–18.

24. Neiger R, Contag SA, Coustan DR. The resolution of preeclampsia related thrombocytopenia. Obstet Gynecol 1991;77:692–699.

25. Romero R, Vizoso J, Emamian M, et al. Clinical significance of liver dysfunction in pregnancy-induced hypertension. Am J Perinatol 1988;5:146–151.

26. Kirshon B, Lee W, Mauer MB, Cotton DB. Effects of low-dose dopamine therapy in the oliguric patient with preeclampsia. Am J Obstet Gynecol 1988;159:604–607.

27. Sibai BM, Mabie BC, Harvey CJ, Gonzalez AR. Pulmonary edema in severe preeclampsia-eclampsia: analysis of thirty-seven consecutive cases. Am J Obstet Gynecol 1987;156:1174–1179.

28. Benedetti TJ, Kates R, Williams V. Hemodynamic observations in severe preeclampsia complicated by pulmonary edema. Am J Obstet Gynecol 1985;152:330–334.

29. Stein L, Bernad JJ, Morissette M, Da Luz P, Weil MH, Shubin H. Pulmonary edema during volume infusion. Circulation 1975;52:483.

30. Benedetti TJ, Quilligan EJ. Cerebral edema in severe preg-

nancy induced hypertension. Am J Obstet Gynecol 1980; 137:860–861.

31. Miller JD. The management of cerebral oedema. Br J Hosp Med 1979;21:152–165.

32. Jouppila P, Jouppila R, Hollmen A, Koivula A. Lumbar epidural analgesia to improve intervillous blood flow during labor in severe preeclampsia. Obstet Gynecol 1982;59: 158–161.

33. Mires GJ, Dempster J, Patel NB, Taylor DJ. Epidural analgesia and its effect on umbilical artery flow velocity waveform patterns in uncomplicated labour and labour complicated by pregnancy-induced hypertension. Eur J Obstet Gynecol Reprod Biol 1990;36:35–41.

34. Connell H, Dalgleish JG, Downing JW. General anaesthesia in mothers with severe pre-eclampsia/eclampsia. Br J Anaesth 1987;59:1375–1380.

35. Benedetti TJ, Cotton DB, Read JC, Miller FC. Hemodynamic observations in severe pre-eclampsia with a flow-directed pulmonary artery catheter. Am J Obstet Gynecol 1980;136:465–470.

36. Cotton DB, Gonik B, Dorman K, Harrist R. Cardiovascular alterations in severe pregnancy-induced hypertension: relationship of central venous pressure to pulmonary capillary wedge pressure. Am J Obstet Gynecol 1985;151: 762–764.

37. Phelan JP, Yurth DA. Severe preeclampsia. I. Peripartum hemodynamic observations. Am J Obstet Gynecol 1982; 144:17–22.

38. Cotton DB, Lee W, Huhta JC, Dorman KF. Hemodynamic profile of severe pregnancy-induced hypertension. Am J Obstet Gynecol 1988;158:523–529.

39. Henderson DW, Vilos GA, Milne KJ, Nichol PM. The role of Swan-Ganz catheterization in severe pregnancy-

induced hypertension. Am J Obstet Gynecol 1984;148:
570–574.

40. Paul RH, Koh KS, Bernstein SG. Changes in fetal heart
    rate: uterine contraction patterns associated with eclamp-
    sia. Am J Obstet Gynecol 1978;130:165.

41. Pritchard JA, Cunningham G, Pritchard SA. The Parkland
    Memorial Hospital protocol for the treatment of eclamp-
    sia: evaluation of 245 cases. Am J Obstet Gynecol 1984;
    148:951.

42. Mabie WC, Ratts TE, Ramanathan KB, Sibai BM. Circu-
    latory congestion in obese hypertensive women: a subset
    of pulmonary edema in pregnancy. Obstet Gynecol 1988;
    72:553–558.

Cardiac Disease

▼　　▼　　▼　　▼　　▼

C ARDIAC DISEASE REMAINS one of the most frequent causes of maternal mortality during pregnancy. As the frequency of rheumatic heart disease has diminished, congenital malformations have become the more common type complicating pregnancy. Preconceptional or early antenatal evaluation of cardiac status, consultation with a cardiologist, and availability of information to the clinician responsible for intrapartum management will facilitate comprehensive care of the patient. The increased risks of pregnancy associated with heart disease depend on the lesion and the patient's baseline cardiac function. The New York Heart Association Classification (Table 2.1) is helpful in predicting maternal outcome. The prediction of maternal mortality may be more accurate when a scheme based on the etiology and anatomy of the cardiac defect is utilized (Table 2.2) (1).

Cardiac disease during the gravid state is influenced by several critical hemodynamic changes, including an increase in blood volume, cardiac output, and heart rate, and a decrease in systemic vascular resistance (2–5). Thus, cardiac patients may have an exacerbation of symptoms and clinical signs that require lifestyle changes during the antenatal period. During the intrapartum period, as a general rule, stroke volume, cardiac

Table 2.1 *New York Heart Association classification*

Class I	Asymptomatic
Class II	Symptoms with more than normal activity
Class III	Symptoms with normal activity
Class IV	Symptoms at bed rest

output, and mean arterial pressure increase, and heart rate decreases, with each contraction when the patient is supine. Maternal positioning, anxiety and pain, and pharmacologic intervention can significantly alter these responses. Immediately following delivery, baseline cardiac output increases by 60% compared to the prelabor output (6–7), and cardiac decompensation remains a significant risk during the first week postpartum.

GENERAL MANAGEMENT PRINCIPLES

The general intrapartum management principles for the cardiac patient are listed in Table 2.3.

Considerations for Delivery

Vaginal delivery may be anticipated in women with cardiac disease, and cesarean section should be reserved for standard obstetric indications. Women with class I or II heart disease may be allowed to go into spontaneous labor at term providing there are no other complicating factors. Regardless of the cardiac lesion, patients should be placed in the left lateral position during labor to maintain preload and reduce hemodynamic fluctuations.

Table 2.2 *Maternal mortality associated with cardiac disease*

Group 1—mortality < 1%

Atrial septal defect

Ventricular septal defect

Patent ductus arteriosus

Pulmonic/tricuspid disease

Tetralogy of Fallot, corrected

Bioprosthetic valve

Mitral stenosis, NYHA class I and II

Group 2—mortality 5–15%

2A

Mitral stenosis, NYHA class III and IV

Aortic stenosis

Coarctation of aorta, without valvular involvement

Uncorrected tetralogy of Fallot

Previous myocardial infarction

Marfan syndrome with normal aorta

2B

Mitral stenosis with atrial fibrillation

Artificial valve

Group 3—mortality 25–50%

Pulmonary hypertension

Coarctation of aorta, with valvular involvement

Marfan's syndrome with aortic involvement

*Modified from Clark SL. Structural cardiac disease in pregnancy. In: Clark SL, Cotton DB, Hankins GDV, Phelan JP, eds. Critical care obstetrics. 2nd ed. Cambridge: Blackwell Scientific Publications, 1991: 115.

Table 2.3 *General intrapartum management principles of the cardiac patient*

Allow spontaneous labor at term (scheduled induction if
   invasive monitoring is needed)

Left lateral positioning

Accurate monitoring of fluid intake and urine output

Adequate pain relief (consider conduction anesthesia)

Oxygen, pulse oximetry, and electrocardiographic monitoring
   as indicated

Invasive hemodynamic monitoring (class III and IV disease)

Shorten second stage of labor

Fluid intake and output, and heart rate and rhythm should be carefully monitored during labor. The selective use of oxygen will reduce the potential for maternal hypoxemia, and noninvasive monitoring can be easily accomplished with pulse oximetry. In addition to pain relief, conduction anesthesia has the benefit of minimizing intrapartum hemodynamic fluctuations. Invasive cardiac monitoring is generally not indicated for patients with class I or II disease, but the requirement for a pulmonary artery catheter should be assessed on an individual basis.

Elective induction may be considered when it is anticipated that a patient with significant disease will require invasive monitoring in an intensive care setting. The same general principles regarding mode of delivery, judicious use of fluid, monitoring of cardiac status, oxygen administration, left lateral positioning, and conduction anesthesia apply to this group of patients. When possible, antepartum consultation with an anesthesiologist will provide the opportunity to evaluate the patient's cardiac status and formulate an intrapartum management plan for pain control. Preload and afterload can be monitored and manipulated most accurately during the intrapartum period via a pulmonary artery catheter and radial arterial line. Assistance with the second stage of labor is recommended since the Valsalva maneuver transiently reduces cardiac output. Blood loss at delivery should be carefully estimated, and it is important to remember that fluid shifts and blood loss are often greater with cesarean section than vaginal delivery.

Invasive hemodynamic monitoring should be considered in any gravida with class III or IV heart disease. However, it is important to remember that the pulmonary artery catheter may not accurately reflect left ventricular function in patients with significant mitral stenosis, severe left ventricular dysfunction, or myocardial infarction. The critical care section (Chapter 9) provides further details regarding the pulmonary artery catheter and hemodynamic parameters for the normal gravida at term.

Anesthesia

Conduction anesthesia has become the preferred method of providing intrapartum pain control for the patient with cardiac disease (8). A regional block minimizes the release of endogenous catecholamines and other neuroendocrine transmitters involved in the stress response, thus reducing hemodynamic fluctuations (9). However, when establishing the regional anesthesia, it is important to avoid the hypotension associated with the loss of sympathetic tone. Careful administration of 1000 mL of crystalloid prior to establishment of the anesthetic will increase the patient's preload and help prevent hypotension.

Ephedrine is considered the agent of choice for the treatment of hypotension associated with regional anesthesia, and it should be available for immediate administration. Ephedrine (5–15 mg given intravenously) acts as an inotrope and chronotrope, increases arterial resistance, and constricts venous capacitance vessels. Phenylephrine (0.2-mg initial intravenous dose; may increase by 0.1–0.2 mg, up to 0.5-mg maximum single dose) is an alternative agent for the treatment of hypotension, but unlike ephedrine, causes partial constriction of placental vessels (9). Although phenylephrine also increases arterial resistance, it has no effect on the venous beds and no significant inotropic or chronotropic effect. Thus, phenylephrine may be a more appropriate choice for patients in whom tachycardia and increased myocardial contractility must be avoided (e.g., patients with mitral and aortic stenosis, coronary artery disease, idiopathic hypertrophic subaortic stenosis, or Eisenmenger's syndrome).

A single-dose spinal technique is relatively contraindicated in patients with significant cardiac disease as hypotension is frequently experienced during establishment of a spinal block. Avoidance of systemic hypotension is crucial for patients with a right-to-left shunt because the decreased blood pressure will only worsen the hemodynamic abnormality. A narcotic epidural is an excellent alternative method that does not affect sympathetic tone and may be particularly effective for patients in whom systemic hypotension must be avoided (e.g., patients with pulmonary hypertension, Eisenmenger's syndrome, or cyanotic heart disease). However, a local injection of lidocaine or a pudendal block may be necessary during the second stage of labor because a narcotic epidural provides minimal perineal anesthesia. Regional anesthesia is typically contraindicated in anticoagulated patients, by the presence of a coagulopathy, or with systemic infection.

Bacterial Endocarditis Prophylaxis

Endocarditis prophylaxis at delivery in patients with structural heart disease remains controversial, and a controlled clinical trial has never been conducted to determine its necessity. Seaworth and Durack (10) suggested that two factors be considered in assessing the need for antibiotic prophylaxis: 1) the underlying cardiac lesion, and 2) the risk of the procedure causing bacteremia. Previous studies demonstrated that bacteremia following vaginal delivery occurs in 1 to 5% of patients (11–14), which is significantly lower than the 60 to 90% incidence associated with dental procedures. The American Heart Association (15) does not recommend prophylaxis for urethral catheterization, uncomplicated vaginal delivery, cesarean section, or sterilization when there is no clinical evidence of infection. In the presence of infection, antibiotic prophylaxis should be administered for these obstetric procedures. In addition, physicians may elect to administer antibiotic prophylaxis to patients with prosthetic heart valves, a history of endocarditis, or surgically constructed systemic-pulmonary shunts even in the setting of low-risk procedures. Antibiotic prophylaxis as recommended by the American Heart Association is listed in Table 2.4. Of note, although cephalosporins are frequently administered for obstetric infection, they are not appropriate prophylaxis against endocarditis since enterococci are not sensitive to these agents.

■ MANAGEMENT OF VALVULAR LESIONS

Mitral Stenosis

Mitral stenosis is the most common valvular lesion encountered during pregnancy and is most frequently the result of rheumatic heart disease. Pregnancy can have a profound, even life-threatening effect on the circulatory system of a woman with mitral stenosis. Maternal mortality ranges from less than 1% for class I or II disease to 4 to 5% for class III or IV disease. The presence of atrial fibrillation further increases this risk, with a maternal mortality rate of 14 to 17%.

The hemodynamic defect is left atrial outflow tract obstruction with decreased left ventricular filling during diastole, a fixed cardiac output, and eventually dilation of the left atrium. Pulmonary congestion and edema may rapidly develop as a result of the increased left atrial and pulmonary capillary wedge pressure (PCWP). With progressive left atrial dilation, the risks of atrial arrhythmias (fibrillation and flutter) and thrombus formation increase significantly. Severe mitral stenosis may result in pulmonary hypertension secondary to long-standing elevation of left atrial pressure.

The intrapartum period represents a high-risk time

Table 2.4 *Endocarditis prophylaxis regimens for genitourinary and gastrointestinal procedures**

Drug	Dosage Regimen
Standard regimen	
Ampicillin, gentamicin, and amoxicillin	Intravenous or intramuscular administration of ampicillin, 2 gm, plus gentamicin, 1.5 mg/kg (not to exceed 80 mg), 30 min before procedure; followed by amoxicillin, 1.5 gm orally 6 hr after initial dose; alternatively, the parenteral regimen may be repeated once 8 hr after initial dose
Ampicillin/amoxicillin/penicillin-allergic patient regimen	
Vancomycin and gentamicin	Intravenous administration of vancomycin, 1 gm over 1 hr plus intravenous or intramuscular administration of gentamicin, 1.5 mg/kg (not to exceed 80 mg), 1 hr before procedure; may be repeated once 8 hr after initial dose
Alternate low-risk patient regimen	
Amoxicillin	3 gm orally, 1 hr before procedure; then 1.5 gm 6 hr after initial dose

*Reprinted by permission from Dajani AS, Bisno AL, Chung KJ, et al. Prevention of bacterial endocarditis: recommendations by the American Heart Association. JAMA 1990;264:2919–2922. Copyright 1990, American Medical Association.

for the gravida with mitral stenosis. Tachycardia, regardless of the etiology, may be a significant contributor to cardiac decompensation as a rapid heart rate decreases left ventricular filling time and results in a further decrease in cardiac output. It has been suggested that beta-blocker therapy (propranolol, 20–40 mg given orally every 6 hours) be considered for any patient with significant mitral stenosis who enters labor with a heart rate faster than 90 beats/minute (16,17). A beta blocker can also be administered intravenously (propranolol, 1–3 mg administered at 1 mg/minute) should sudden tachycardia develop during labor. Conduction anesthesia is an excellent method to reduce the pain and anxiety of labor, which contribute significantly to an increased heart rate. The second stage of labor may be shortened by operative vaginal delivery to minimize the risk of tachycardia associated with bearing down to deliver the infant.

Atrial fibrillation represents an additional complication when mitral stenosis is accompanied by left atrial dilation. A patient with preexisting fibrillation should be continued on antiarrhythmic therapy throughout labor. These patients are usually placed on full-dose heparin to prevent thrombus formation in a dilated atrium with poor contractility. The management of the heparinized patient can be found under a separate section of this text. New-onset atrial fibrillation during labor should be treated with digitalis in the hemodynamically stable patient or cardioversion in the event of hemodynamic instability (18).

Invasive monitoring with a pulmonary artery catheter should be anticipated for patients with class III or IV disease. Assessing central venous pressure (CVP) is not an accurate method of monitoring patients with mitral stenosis because it correlates poorly with PCWP (16). Additionally, it must be remembered that the PCWP does not adequately estimate the left ventricular diastolic filling pressure in patients with mitral stenosis. Thus, a falsely elevated PCWP should be anticipated.

The immediate postpartum period seems to be a particularly hazardous time for women with mitral stenosis. Rapid volume shifts due to the release of vena caval obstruction, autotransfusion of blood from the uteroplacental circulation, and decreased vascular capacitance result in an increased preload. Patients with a fixed cardiac output as in mitral stenosis cannot accommodate this increase in preload, and acute hydrostatic pulmonary edema may ensue rapidly. Close attention to fluid intake and output is important to prevent iatrogenic fluid overload. Careful diuresis with furosemide may be required to decrease the preload, and is best guided by invasive hemodynamic parameters. However, excessive diuresis must be avoided since patients with mitral stenosis depend on a normal to high-normal PCWP to maintain adequate left ventricular diastolic filling pressure.

Mitral Insufficiency

Mitral insufficiency is generally well tolerated during pregnancy unless severe regurgitation and left ventricular dysfunction are present. Unlike mitral stenosis, rheumatic heart disease is less commonly associated with this condition. Mitral regurgitation in older women may be the result of hypertension, myocardial ischemia or disease, or infectious endocarditis.

The hemodynamic aberration is a reflux of blood from the left ventricle into the atrium during systole with gradual left atrial dilation and left ventricular hypertrophy. The decrease in systemic vascular resistance associated with pregnancy generally favors an increase in the forward flow of blood with less backward flow from the left ventricle to the atrium. Women with mitral insufficiency tend to tolerate mild tachycardia much better than women with a stenotic mitral valve. Patients with mild to moderate insufficiency and normal left ventricular function may be managed according to the general guidelines previously discussed.

Patients having severe insufficiency with left ventricular dysfunction and possibly pulmonary hypertension are at a significantly higher risk of complications during labor. If atrial fibrillation is present, antiarrhythmic therapy and anticoagulation will be required to decrease the risk of systemic embolization. Invasive monitoring to optimize preload, afterload, and cardiac output should be strongly considered during labor. Conduction anesthesia will aid in reducing afterload but must be carefully administered in a patient with secondary pulmonary hypertension.

Mitral Valve Prolapse

Mitral valve prolapse (MVP) occurs in approximately 17% of women, and whether this is a normal variant or congenital anomaly is debatable. The majority of women with MVP are asymptomatic, but some individuals experience palpitations, chest pain, and dysrhythmia that require treatment with a beta-blocking agent. When a dysrhythmia is present in spite of beta-blocker administration, conventional antiarrhythmic therapy is required.

No special management is required during labor for women with asymptomatic prolapse, and although controversial, antibiotic prophylaxis is not recommended for women with MVP in the absence of a systolic murmur (19). Women with symptomatic prolapse should continue their antepartum medication regimen (usually propranolol) throughout labor. Because propranolol has been associated with intrauterine growth restriction (20), the clinician should be aware of the fetus's estimated weight. Continuous fetal monitoring should be employed in this circumstance given the increased risk of intrapartum fetal distress experienced by the small fetus. Because alterations in fetal heart rate reactivity have been reported in women taking propranolol, additional intrapartum fetal evaluation may be needed to ensure fetal well-being. Pediatric evaluation of the newborn may be required as postdelivery hypoglycemia and bradycardia have occurred in infants exposed to this agent. When a woman has significant regurgitation associated with MVP, the principles outlined for mitral insufficiency apply.

Aortic Stenosis

Isolated aortic stenosis is usually congenital in nature, but additional lesions are frequently present when there is a rheumatic etiology. The major hemodynamic problem is the maintenance of cardiac output, which is relatively fixed when the stenosis is severe. During pregnancy, hypervolemia increases left ventricular filling pressure and favors increased cardiac output. Patients with a valvular gradient exceeding 100 mm Hg appear to be at the highest risk for sudden death due to myocardial ischemia (21). Because of the pressure gradient across the aortic valve, left ventricular hypertrophy develops slowly over time.

The time of greatest risk for patients with aortic stenosis is during labor and delivery or with pregnancy termination. Invasive hemodynamic monitoring is recommended for accurate management of fluid status in patients with class III or IV disease. Easterling et al (22) suggested placement of a pulmonary artery catheter on the evening before induction, to optimize preload and afterload. Adequate preload must be ensured in order for the left ventricle to maintain cardiac output, and hypotension associated with regional anesthesia or hemorrhage may result in decreased output. However, a small increase in intravascular volume may result in pulmonary edema secondary to elevated filling pressures in a patient with a fixed cardiac output. Tachycardia must be avoided because it reduces diastolic filling and coronary perfusion with resultant ischemia.

As with other cardiac lesions, careful use of regional anesthesia can decrease the tachycardia associated with the pain and anxiety of labor. An assisted second stage of labor is indicated to minimize the effects of the Valsalva maneuver. Patients with aortic stenosis require careful monitoring during the initial 24 hours after delivery because they are at risk of developing pulmonary edema secondary to the autotransfusion that occurs postpartum.

Aortic Insufficiency

Aortic insufficiency is most frequently the result of rheumatic heart disease, with regurgitant blood flow into the left ventricle during diastole. Left ventricular hypertrophy may ensue with long-standing disease. It is important to exclude a mitral valvular lesion, as these are often associated with aortic insufficiency. Pregnancy does not usually cause any difficulties for the woman with aortic insufficiency. As heart rate increases with gestation, diastole is shortened and results in less backward flow into the left ventricle. Additionally, the physiologic reduction in afterload during pregnancy also leads to a reduction in regurgitation. Pharmacologic afterload reduction may, however, be required if pulmonary edema develops in a patient with severe aortic insufficiency.

Prosthetic Heart Valve

The care of a patient who has undergone surgical correction of congenital or acquired valvular heart disease merits consideration of several issues. Patients with a prosthetic heart valve are at increased risk of systemic emboli, anticoagulation complications, bacterial endocarditits, and valvular dysfunction. The maternal risks during pregnancy do not appear to differ with the type of replaced valve (23).

The type of valve has implications regarding the need for anticoagulation, with a tissue valve eliminating this requirement. However, compared with a mechanical valve, the tissue valve carries a higher likelihood of subsequent reoperation for replacement. Patients with a mechanical valve require lifelong therapeutic anticoagulation to minimize the risk of embolization. During pregnancy, subcutaneous heparin adjusted to achieve an activated partial thromboplastin time (aPTT) of 1.5 to 2.0 times the patient's baseline value is the therapy of choice. A complete discussion of the intrapartum management of the anticoagulated patient can be found under a separate section of this text.

Patients with a prosthetic valve are at risk for bacterial endocarditis and valvular dysfunction regardless of valve type. The current antibiotic recommendations are addressed at the beginning of this chapter and all patients should receive prophylaxis accordingly. Cardiac echocardiography is an excellent noninvasive method for the evaluation of valvular function and should be performed whenever a patient demonstrates symptoms or signs of dysfunction during the intrapartum or postpartum period.

■ CONGENITAL HEART DISEASE

Left-to-Right Shunts

Atrial Septal Defect: Ostium secundum defects are the most common congenital cardiac lesions encountered in pregnancy. Most women with an atrial septal defect (ASD) are asymptomatic and tolerate pregnancy without cardiac complications. Women older than 35 years with an uncorrected large ASD are at risk of having Eisenmenger's syndrome, which carries a significantly higher mortality.

The decreased peripheral resistance in the gravid woman may actually decrease the left-to-right shunt of an ASD. However, the hypervolemia of pregnancy may increase the left-to-right shunt through the ASD and thus the work of the right ventricle, resulting in right-sided heart failure. An ASD is rarely associated with congestive heart failure but this has been reported (24–26). A small percentage of patients develop an atrial arrhythmia (most frequently fibrillation) requiring medical therapy. In the absence of Eisenmenger's syndrome, labor and delivery may be conducted as previously outlined without any considerations specific to ASDs.

Ventricular Septal Defect: Ventricular septal defects (VSDs) range from small isolated lesions that pose no special risks during pregnancy to large defects accompanied by Eisenmenger's syndrome and significant maternal risk. Large VSDs are more frequently associated with aortic insufficiency, congestive failure, arrhythmias, and the development of pulmonary hypertension. Once pulmonary hypertension (Eisenmenger's syndrome) is present, pregnancy will worsen the right-to-left shunt because systemic vascular resistance decreases without a corresponding decrease in pulmonary artery pressures. Thus, pregnancy will worsen the patient's hypoxia by increasing the shunting of blood away from the lungs. VSDs may also occur in association with other congenital cardiac lesions such as transposition of the great vessels, tetralogy of Fallot, and coarctation of the aorta.

Labor and delivery are generally well tolerated by patients with an uncomplicated VSD. As with other cardiac patients, careful attention to lateral positioning, fluid management, pain relief, oxygen administration, and fetal monitoring is important. Women with Eisenmenger's syndrome require intensive intrapartum monitoring, which is discussed subsequently.

Patent Ductus Arteriosus: Few women reach childbearing age with a patent ductus arteriosus (PDA) as most are now repaired during early childhood. A patient who has a small PDA is generally asymptomatic and has an excellent prognosis during pregnancy. However, a large patent ductus is associated with a high-pressure high-flow left-to-right shunt, and Eisenmenger's syndrome may develop secondary to the increased flow through the low-resistance pulmonary circulation. In the presence of pulmonary hypertension, the prognosis for a PDA significantly worsens and maternal mortality reaches 50%.

Right-to-Left Shunt

Primary Pulmonary Hypertension and Eisenmenger's Syndrome: Primary pulmonary hypertension can be identified when clinical, radiographic, and invasive hemodynamic data support arterial hypertension within the pulmonary vasculature. By definition, this condition has no clear identifiable etiology. Eisenmenger's syndrome develops when an unrepaired congenital left-to-right shunt results in progressive secondary pulmonary hypertension. The maternal mortality rate in the presence of pulmonary hypertension has been reported to be 30% to 50%. It appears that mortality is higher when Eisenmenger's syndrome is associated with a VSD than an ASD or PDA, and cesarean section carries a higher risk than vaginal delivery (27).

As with many other cardiac lesions, the intrapartum and early postpartum periods are the times of highest risk of decompensation and sudden death in patients with pulmonary hypertension. Induction of labor in an intensive care setting should be coordinated with the patient's cardiologist and an obstetric anesthesiologist to facilitate obstetric, cardiac, and pain management. There is no evidence of any harmful effect of prostaglandin gel for cervical ripening, and limited information suggests that oxytocin has no effect on the right-to-left shunt of Eisenmenger's syndrome (28). Cesarean section should be reserved for standard obstetric indications, and vaginal delivery remains the mode of choice. The second stage of labor may be assisted with forceps or vacuum delivery.

Continuous pulse oximetry and an arterial line may assist in monitoring the patient with pulmonary hypertension during labor. The immediate availability of information offered by an arterial line is advantageous in the event of acute hypotension requiring treatment. Oxygen is considered the pulmonary vasodilator of choice (28) and should be administered throughout labor and delivery. Continuous electronic fetal monitoring should be employed given the low baseline maternal oxygen pressure and increased risk of intrauterine growth restriction.

In Eisenmenger's syndrome, as the pulmonary vasculature hypertrophies and vascular resistance increases, reversal of the shunt or bidirectional flow through the preexisting defect (ASD, VSD, or PDA) occurs. During pregnancy, systemic vascular resistance decreases and the degree of right-to-left shunting increases. Pulmonary perfusion decreases and hypoxemia increases as a result of the worsening shunt. If right-sided heart filling pressure is suddenly reduced (as with hypovolemia, hemorrhage, or hypotension with conduction anesthesia), perfusion of the pulmonary arterial bed may be insufficient and profound hypoxemia and sudden death may occur. Additional causes of death in patients with Eisenmenger's syndrome include embolism, myocardial infarction, and arrhythmias.

Great care must be taken when establishing and maintaining vascular access due to the risk of paradoxical embolism in patients with a right-to-left shunt. Thrombi, air, or septic emboli may pass from the peripheral to central circulation because the lungs are unable to filter blood as normally occurs. It is recommended that to minimize this risk, air filters be utilized for all intravenous lines (29).

The need for invasive monitoring of patients with Eisenmenger's syndrome during labor has been debated. Unfortunately, the placement of a Swan-Ganz catheter may be complicated or prohibited by the patient's underlying cardiac pathology. Those who favor its use believe that the pulmonary artery catheter allows accurate assessment of the patient's preload and correction of early changes in volume status and cardiac output. Because hypovolemia and hypotension are life threatening in Eisenmenger's syndrome, it is recommended that preload be maintained with a margin of safety in the event of excessive blood loss at delivery (30). Diuresis should always be undertaken with extreme caution. Opponents of use of the pulmonary artery catheter believe that the risks associated with placement (arrhythmia, emboli to the systemic circulation, pulmonary artery rupture) outweigh the limited information available regarding preload and cardiac output. The PCWP and thermodilution techniques are unreliable in patients with pulmonary hypertension due to the effects of hypertrophied pulmonary arteries and shunting, respectively.

Although the week following delivery represents the most frequent time of death for patients with Eisenmenger's syndrome, delayed sudden death has occurred as late as 6 weeks following delivery (27). The etiology is not always discernible, but thromboembolism is responsible for a significant proportion of deaths. Prophylactic heparinization may be considered during labor, delivery, and the postpartum period, but the benefits have not been clearly shown, given the limited number of patients in this clinical situation.

Tetralogy of Fallot: Tetralogy of Fallot is a cyanotic congenital heart disease consisting of a VSD, overriding aorta, pulmonic stenosis, and right ventricular hypertrophy. The majority of women born with this condition will have undergone surgical repair during childhood and generally do not incur any increased risks with pregnancy. However, some patients may have a clinically significant conduction defect or arrhythmia in spite of surgical correction of the VSD and pulmonary stenosis. Patients requiring antiarrhythmic therapy should continue receiving the agent intrapartum, and continuous cardiac monitoring can be considered to detect any acute change in the patient's status.

A woman with an uncorrected tetralogy of Fallot is at significantly increased risk during pregnancy. The normal reduction in systemic vascular resistance with pregnancy only worsens the right-to-left shunt and further decreases pulmonary blood flow. Several factors have been associated with a poor prognosis for patients with tetralogy during pregnancy (Table 2.5) (29).

The intrapartum management of patients with an

Table 2.5 *Poor prognostic factors for gravidas with tetralogy of Fallot*

Hematocrit > 65%

History of syncope or congestive failure

Evidence of right ventricular strain on electrocardiogram

Cardiomegaly

Right ventricular pressure > 120 mm Hg

Oxygen saturation < 80%

---

uncorrected tetralogy of Fallot is similar to the care of patients with pulmonary hypertension. Maintenance of preload and right-sided end-diastolic volume is critical to adequate hemodynamic function. Conduction anesthesia should be administered with care to avoid hypotension, and a shortened second stage of labor through the use of forceps or vacuum may be considered. Blood loss at the time of delivery must be carefully monitored, and replacement with blood products should not be delayed in the event of hemorrhage. The patient with tetralogy of Fallot should be observed closely during the initial postpartum period as this remains a high-risk time during which complications may arise.

Coarctation of the Aorta: Coarctation of the aorta may be found as an isolated lesion or associated with other malformations including VSD, PDA, aortic stenosis, or aortic insufficiency due to a bicuspid valve. Isolated hypertension in the upper extremities and decreased femoral pulses are suggestive of this lesion. If the diagnosis is made prior to conception, surgical correction is recommended before attempting pregnancy.

Patients with surgically corrected coarctation of the aorta or an isolated lesion without aneurysmal dilation and class I or II heart disease generally tolerate pregnancy without difficulty. However, women with uncorrected coarctation of the aorta have a fixed stroke volume. They are at risk of a dissecting hematoma of the aorta beyond the constriction or in the intercostal arteries, and endocarditis when an anomalous aortic valve is present. Left ventricular hypertrophy may be present as a result of the long-standing obstruction. Coarctation may also be associated with a congenital intracranial aneurysm of the circle of Willis.

During labor, careful attention to volume status is important. Hypovolemia may reduce perfusion pressure distal to the uncorrected lesion, but volume overload may result in congestive heart failure and pulmonary edema in patients with an uncorrected or complex lesion. Hypertension should be controlled to decrease the risk of vascular rupture which is secondary to an increased heart rate and contractility. Beta blockers have the potential advantage of less tachycardia than other antihypertensive agents. However, bradycardia is not well tolerated in the presence of a fixed stroke volume, as heart rate primarily determines cardiac output. Additional anesthesia-based recommendations include maintenance of a normal to elevated systemic vascular resistance by using "light" anesthesia during delivery in the patient with significant coarctation (31). This will avoid hypotension due to an uncompensated iatrogenic reduction in systemic vascular resistance. Likewise, left ventricular filling pressure should be maintained by avoidance of hypovolemia or reductions in venous return.

■ OTHER CARDIAC DISEASES

Marfan's Syndrome

Marfan's syndrome is inherited as an autosomal dominant trait that has variable expressivity. The connective tissue weakness of this disorder results in ocular, cardiovascular, pulmonary, and skeletal abnormalities. The vascular system is affected by cystic medial necrosis of the aorta, aortic regurgitation, and dissecting aneurysms. Pregnancy apparently increases the risk of these cardiovascular complications. MVP occurs in most patients with Marfan's syndrome and is secondary to redundant chordae tendineae and mitral leaflets. Antenatal echocardiography should be performed to assess cardiac function and determine the presence or absence of aortic root dilation. Women with an aortic root diameter more than 40 mm reportedly have a pregnancy-related mortality rate approaching 50% versus a rate of 5% when the aortic root is not dilated (32).

The increased cardiac output during pregnancy may cause worsening of aortic insufficiency and increased aortic root dilation. During pregnancy and labor, blood pressure must be carefully controlled to minimize shear stress. Administration of a beta blocker (propranolol, 2–5 mg every 4 hours) may decrease the pulsatile pressure on the aortic wall and reduce the risk of acute dissection of the aorta. An arterial line can be of assistance in monitoring blood pressure, particularly if vasoactive agents are required.

Epidural anesthesia will provide relief of pain and anxiety, and aid in maintaining a normal heart rate. The Valsalva maneuver should be avoided, and outlet forceps or vacuum delivery is indicated. Cesarean section should be reserved for standard obstetric indications. Since methylergonovine maleate (Methergine) can cause maternal tachycardia, 15-methylprostaglandin $F_{2\alpha}$ should be considered the second-line agent (after oxytocion) for the treatment of uterine atony. Blood pressure and cardiac status must be carefully followed during the postpartum period, given the continued increase in cardiac output that occurs after delivery.

Idiopathic Hypertrophic Subaortic Stenosis

Idiopathic hypertrophic subaortic stenosis is inherited as an autosomal dominant disorder with variable penetrance. Patients may not manifest any evidence of the condition until the second or third decade of life. The left ventricular septum is primarily involved, and the septal hypertrophy results in left ventricular outflow obstruction and secondary mitral regurgitation. The increased plasma volume of pregnancy is well tolerated as the maintenance of preload is important for left ventricular filling. Although data are limited, maternal and fetal outcome appear to be favorable for these patients (33).

During the intrapartum period, avoidance of hypotension and tachycardia is important as both of these will result in decreased left-sided filling pressure and worsen the outflow obstruction. The patient should be in the left lateral position during labor because this will prevent aortocaval compression. In the symptomatic patient (dyspnea, syncope, angina, palpitations, and arrhythmia), a beta blocker will reduce myocardial contractility and heart rate, thus allowing greater diastolic filling time. Calcium channel blockers (oral verapamil, 120–480 mg/day in divided doses) also can be effective treatment for the symptomatic patient. Volume status should be carefully observed during labor.

Pain management with epidural anesthesia may aid in the reduction of tachycardia associated with the pain and anxiety of labor. Ephedrine should be avoided since it will increase the occlusive effect of this lesion by virtue of reflex tachycardia. Hypotension related to regional anesthesia placement may be corrected with phenylephrine, 1 to 10 mg intravenously titrated to pressor response. Having the patient perform the Valsalva maneuver during the second stage of labor will reduce venous return, and an operative vaginal delivery may be considered. Cardiac monitoring should be continued for 24 hours following delivery.

Coronary Artery Disease and Myocardial Infarction

Coronary artery disease is uncommon in women of reproductive age, and myocardial infarction during pregnancy is rare. An ischemic event in pregnancy may be precipitated by atherosclerosis, coronary artery spasm, embolic phenomeneon, preeclampsia, cardiac arrhythmia, or substance abuse, particularly cocaine. Hankins et al (34) reviewed 68 gravidas who had a myocardial infarction. Of interest, only 13% of these women had a known history of coronary artery disease, and two thirds of the infarctions occurred during the third trimester. The 45% mortality rate for an infarction occurring in the third trimester of pregnancy was much higher than the 23% observed for a first- or second-trimester event. In addition, the mortality rate was increased when delivery occurred within 2 weeks of the infarction.

Women with known myocardial disease should have an antenatal 12-lead electrocardiogram (ECG) to establish their baseline and an echocardiogram to determine left ventricular function. Patients with stable disease may undergo delivery electively when fetal lung maturity is achieved. Although there is limited experience with this group of patients, cesarean section has not been shown to confer any benefit (34). A patient undergoing induction of labor should be placed in an intensive care setting with a cardiologist and anesthesiologist actively involved in her intrapartum care. Placement of a pulmonary artery catheter prior to labor will allow optimization of preload, afterload, and cardiac output. It is important to avoid tachycardia whenever possible as heart rate is one of the major determinants of myocardial oxygen demand. Therefore, adequate analgesia to prevent tachycardia related to pain should be ensured throughout the intrapartum period via intravenous morphine or careful administration of a regional block. A forceps or vacuum delivery will diminish the work of the second stage of labor.

If a patient has chest pain, shortness of breath, or signs of congestive failure during labor, the patient must be evaluated for myocardial ischemia without delay. Serial 12-lead ECG can be compared to the patient's antenatal tracing and continuous cardiac monitoring instituted. A baseline arterial blood gas analysis will provide information regarding the patient's degree of hypoxemia and acid-base balance. Laboratory evaluation including serum electrolyte measurements, blood urea nitrogen (BUN) and creatinine determinations, glucose measurement, urinalysis, and liver function studies can be obtained as indicated.

Serum creatinine kinase (CK) and its isoenzymes are routinely measured in nonpregnant patients suspected of having a myocardial infarction. Myocardium normally contains approximately 80% CK-MB and 20% CK-MM; an elevation of the MB fraction is consistent with an infarction. However, mild increases in total CK and CK-MB have been demonstrated in healthy gravidas during the intrapartum and postpartum periods, using a sensitive immunochemical assay (35). This may be explained by the leaking of CK-MB from placental and myometrial tissue into maternal serum during uterine contractions. Thus, these enzyme measurements should be carefully interpreted in the context of the entire clinical picture.

The initial steps in the management of a patient with a suspected myocardial infarction include adequate analgesia, oxygenation, prevention of arrhythmia, and minimizing myocardial damage. A cardiologist and the intensive care unit team should be consulted once initial treatment measures have been instituted. In the event of acute ischemia, it appears that delivery of the fetus is best avoided unless there is evidence of fetal distress or maternal death is imminent. Generally, it is advisable to make every effort to stabilize the maternal condition prior to undertaking delivery of the fetus.

High-flow oxygen should be administered as myocardial oxygen supply depends on arterial oxygen content. Intravenous administration of morphine sulfate (2–4 mg every 5 minutes to desired effect) decreases the pain associated with ischemia and reduces anxiety. Additionally, it may lower arterial pressure through arteriolar and venous dilation. Nitroglycerin is a vasodilator that dilates the coronary arteries, the peripheral arteries, and particularly the veins. Sublingual nitroglycerin, 0.3 mg administered every 5 minutes to a maximum of three doses, will reduce preload and afterload, and decrease chest pain. Patients must be observed for adverse reactions including hypotension and bradycardia, and nitroglycerin should be avoided in patients with a systolic blood pressure less than 100 mm Hg. The risk of subsequent cardiac arrhythmia is reduced through the intravenous administration of lidocaine (1.0–1.4-mg/kg initial dose followed with a continuous infusion of 1–4 mg/min).

Thrombolytic therapy has played an increasingly important role in the management of acute myocardial infarction, but information regarding its use in pregnant women is limited. The use of these agents is generally limited to life-threatening situations. Complications, including maternal bleeding and premature labor, have been reported (36). Full-dose heparin therapy is indicated in the setting of significant ventricular dyskinesis or a ventricular aneurysm.

Decisions regarding delivery must be individualized, but it is ideally delayed for at least 2 weeks following the ischemic event. Evidence regarding a preferred mode of delivery is scant; there appears to be no difference in maternal mortality between those undergoing vaginal and those having cesarean delivery. However, the largest reported series (34) included only 68 patients and spanned many decades, making firm recommendations difficult given our current state of advanced medical capabilities.

Peripartum Cardiomyopathy

Peripartum cardiomyopathy (PPCM) develops in the last month of pregnancy or during the first 6 months post-partum in a woman without a history of cardiac disease. Patients typically present with a gradual onset of increasing fatigue, dyspnea, paroxysmal nocturnal dyspnea, and pulmonary or peripheral edema. Physical examination reveals signs of congestive heart failure including jugular venous distention, pulmonary rales, and an S_3 gallop. Cardiomegaly and pulmonary edema are seen on chest radiographs, and ECG often shows left atrial and ventricular dilation. Echocardiography should be performed to objectively characterize left ventricular function. The diagnosis of PPCM is one of exclusion, and a thorough evaluation to exclude other causes should be performed at the time of initial presentation.

Admission laboratory studies for the patient with PPCM may include determining the hemoglobin/hematocrit; performing a blood type and screen; measuring electrolyte, BUN, creatinine, and digoxin levels; and performing coagulation studies. Many patients have been placed on digoxin, a diuretic, and heparin at the time of diagnosis. In addition to hypokalemia, women with PPCM seem more prone to become digoxin toxic on usual dosage regimens. Digoxin should be continued throughout the intrapartum period, given with sips of water at its usual dosage and interval or converted to its intravenous counterpart. The management of a heparinized patient is outlined in Chapter 7.

The risk of hypotension, pulmonary edema, thromboembolism, hypoxia, myocardial ischemia, and arrhythmias make the intrapartum and postpartum periods dangerous times for the gravida with PPCM. General measures such as left lateral positioning, oxygen administration with monitoring by pulse oximetry, adequate pain control, and continuous fetal monitoring remain important in the intrapartum care of these women. It is crucial to avoid hypotension and tachycardia as these can decrease left ventricular diastolic filling time and coronary artery perfusion.

Placement of a pulmonary artery catheter provides accurate hemodynamic information regarding preload (PCWP), afterload (systemic vascular resistance), and cardiac output. However, PCWP may not accurately reflect left ventricular filling pressure in the presence of severe dysfunction of this chamber. The goal of therapy during labor is to maximize cardiac output while maintaining the lowest possible PCWP. If inotropic support is required, dopamine will exert a beta-1 effect at a dose of 5 to 10 μg/kg/minute. Alternatively, dobutamine is a selective beta-1 agonist and results in less tachycardia than dopamine. Clark et al (37) detailed the use of a ventricular function curve in healthy term gravidas whereby left ventricular stroke work index is plotted against PCWP (Figure 2.1). With this graphic model, left ventricular function can then be optimized, specific for pregnancy, by diuresis, volume expansion, or inotropic support.

Vaginal delivery with an assisted second stage is the preferred method of delivery in the absence of an obstet-

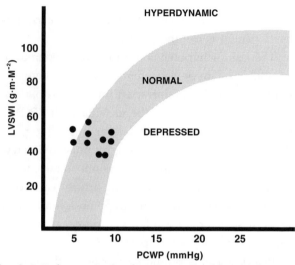

Fig. 2.1 *Left ventricular function in healthy third-trimester pregnant women. (From Clark et al, Am J Obstet Gynecol 1989;161:1440.)*

ric indication requiring cesarean delivery. Carefully administered epidural anesthesia offers the advantage of afterload reduction and minimizes tachycardia related to pain. Postpartum hemodynamic monitoring should be continued for 48 hours because cardiac output continues to increase after delivery and intravascular volume shifts can result in pulmonary edema.

■ REFERENCES

1. Clark SL. Structural cardiac disease in pregnancy. In: Clark SL, Cotton DB, Phelan JP, eds. Critical care obstetrics. 2nd ed. Cambridge: Blackwell Scientific Publications, 1991:115.

2. Scott DE. Anemia during pregnancy. Obstet Gynecol Annu 1972;1:219.

3. Pritchard JA. Changes in the blood volume during pregnancy and delivery. Anesthesiology 1965;26:393.

4. Wilson M, Morganti AA, Zervodakis I, et al. Blood pressure, the renin-aldosterone system, and sex steroids throughout normal pregnancy. Am J Med 1980;68:97.

5. Clark SL, Cotton DB, Lee W, et al. Central hemodynamic assessment of normal term pregnancy. Am J Obstet Gynecol 1989;161:1439.

6. Ueland K, Hansen JM. Maternal cardiovascular hemodynamics. III. Labor and delivery under local and caudal anesthesia. Am J Obstet Gynecol 1969;103:8.

7. Kjeldsen J. Hemodynamic investigations during labor and delivery. Acta Obstet Gynecol Scand Suppl 1979;89:1.

8. Yeager MP. Regional anesthesia for the patient with heart disease. Pro: regional anesthesia is preferable to general anesthesia for the patient with heart disease. J Cardiothorac Anesth 1989;3:793.

9. Ralston DH, Shnider SM, deLorimier AA. Effects of equipotent ephedrine, metaraminol, mephentermine and methoxamine on uterine blood flow in the pregnant ewe. Anesthesiology 1974;40:345.

10. Seaworth BJ, Durack DT. Infective endocarditis in obstetric and gynecologic practice. Am J Obstet Gynecol 1986; 154:180–188.

11. Redleaf PD, Fadell EJ. Bacteremia during parturition. JAMA 1959;169:1284.

12. McCormack WM, Rosner B, Lee Y-H, Rankin JS, Lin J-S. Isolation of genital mycoplasmas from blood obtained shortly after vaginal delivery. Lancet 1975;1:596.

13. Sugrue D, Blake S, Troy P, MacDonald D. Antibiotic prophylaxis against infective endocarditis after normal delivery—is it necessary? Br Heart J 1980;44:499.

14. Baker TH, Hubbell R. Reappraisal of asymptomatic puerperal bacteremia. Am J Obstet Gynecol 1967;97:575.

15. Dajani AS, Bisno AL, Chung KJ, et al. Prevention of bacterial endocarditis. Recommendations by the American Heart Association. JAMA 1990;264:2919–2922.

16. Clark SL, Phelan JP, Greenspoon J, Aldahl D, Horenstein J. Labor and delivery in the presence of mitral stenosis: central hemodynamic observations. Am J Obstet Gynecol 1985;152:984–988.

17. Al Kasab SM, Sabag T, Al Zaibag M, et al. β-Adrenergic receptor blockade in the management of pregnant women with mitral stenosis. Am J Obstet Gynecol 1990;163:37–40.

18. Schroeder JS, Harrison DC. Repeated cardioversion during pregnancy: treatment of refractory paroxysmal atrial tachycardia during three successive pregnancies. Am J Cardiol 1971;27:445.

19. Shabetai R. Cardiac diseases. In: Creasy RK, Resnik R, eds. Maternal-fetal medicine: principles and practice. 3rd ed. Philadelphia: WB Saunders Company, 1994:768.

20. Redmond GP. Propranolol and fetal growth retardation. Semin Perinatol 1982;6:142–147.

21. Arias F, Pineda J. Aortic stenosis and pregnancy. J Reprod Med 1978;20:229.

22. Easterling TR, Chadwick HS, Otto CM, Benedetti TJ. Aortic stenosis in pregnancy. Obstet Gynecol 1988;72:113–118.

23. McAnulty JH, Blair N, Walance C, Ueland K. Prosthetic heart valves and pregnancy: maternal and infant outcome. J Am Coll Cardiol 1986;7:171A.

24. Mendelson CL. Cardiac disease in pregnancy. Philadelphia: FA Davis Company, 1960:151.

25. Neilson G, Galea EG, Blunt A. Congenital heart disease and pregnancy. Med J Aust 1970;30:1086.

26. Schaefer G, Arditi LI, Solomon HA, et al. Congenital heart disease and pregnancy. Clin Obstet Gynecol 1968;11:1048.

27. Gleicher N, Midwall J, Hochberger D, et al. Eisenmenger's syndrome and pregnancy. Obstet Gynecol Surv 1979;34: 721.

28. Midwall J, Jaffin H, Herman MV, Kupersmith J. Shunt flow and pulmonary hemodynamics during labor and delivery in the Eisenmenger syndrome. Am J Cardiol 1978;42:299–303.

29. Patton DE, Lee W, Cotton DB, et al. Cyanotic maternal heart disease in pregnancy. Obstet Gynecol Surv 1990;45: 594–600.

30. Clark SL. Labor and delivery in the patient with structural cardiac disease. Clin Perinatol 1986;13:695.

31. Mangano DT. Anesthesia for the pregnant cardiac patient. In: Shnider SM, Levinson G, eds. Anesthesia for obstetrics. Baltimore: Williams & Wilkins, 1987:345–381.

32. Pyeritz RE. Maternal and fetal complications of pregnancy in Marfan syndrome. Am J Med 1981;71:784.

33. Oakley GDG, McGarry K, Limb DG, et al. Management of pregnancy in patients with hypertrophic cardiomyopathy. BMJ 1979;1:1749.

34. Hankins GDV, Wendel GD, Leveno KJ, Stoneham J. Myocardial infarction during pregnancy: a review. Obstet Gynecol 1985;65:139–146.

35. Leiserowitz GS, Evans AT, Samuels SJ, Omand K, Kost GJ. Creatine kinase and its MB isoenzyme in the third trimester and the peripartum period. J Reprod Med 1992;37: 910–916.

36. Pfeifer GW. The use of thrombolytic therapy in obstetrics and gynecology. Aus Ann Med Suppl 1970;28.

37. Clark SL, Cotton DB, Lee W, et al. Central hemodynamic assessment of normal term pregnancy. Am J Obstet Gynecol 1989;161:1439–1442.

Pulmonary Disease

▼   ▼   ▼   ▼   ▼

■ ASTHMA

Asthma is defined as respiratory compromise due to a reversible airway obstruction. It can be triggered by a variety of precipitating factors, including those of an immunologic, infective, or emotional basis. Between 0.1 and 2.0% of pregnant women have a history of asthma, the prevalence depending on the stringency of the original diagnosis (1–3). Pregnancy does not increase the frequency or severity of asthma in the majority of patients. Conversely, the physiologic and anatomic alterations in respiratory function associated with normal pregnancy may compromise the complicated asthmatic with borderline respiratory reserve. The goal of antepartum care of the pregnant woman with asthma is to achieve optimal control with a minimum of medications. The patient with poorly controlled asthma has an increased risk of intrapartum exacerbation with its associated complications, including hypoxemia, pneumonia, and respiratory failure.

Expectant management and spontaneous labor at term can be anticipated for most patients with asthma. When induction of labor is required for obstetric indications, cervical ripening with prostaglandin E_2 gel is safe, as there have been no reports of bronchoconstriction associated with its use in the asthmatic. Prostaglandin $F_{2\alpha}$, however, may result in bronchospasm when the agent is used in the setting of second-trimester termination of pregnancy (4). Oxytocin has no recognized adverse effects on asthma.

When a patient with asthma is admitted during labor, a peak expiratory flow rate (PEFR) should be determined (Table 3.1). This testing can be easily performed at the bedside with a portable peak flow meter. Objective measures are desirable because the patient's and physician's perceptions of asthma severity are often inaccurate (5). Repeat testing may be performed subsequently in the symptomatic patient, or to follow the clinical response to bronchodilator therapy. The normal nonpregnant range of PEFR is 380 to 550 L/minute, and this closely approximates the forced expiratory volume of air in 1 second (FEV_1). A patient's antepartum PEFR can be utilized as a general guideline to assess the stability of her disease state. An intrapartum PEFR of at least 80% of the baseline value suggests the patient's asthma is well controlled.

In patients taking antepartum medications, the regimen should be continued throughout labor, delivery, and the postpartum period. Inhaled steroids or beta mimetics should be administered at their usual dosage and interval. Oral medications can be administered during labor, although alterations in gastrointestinal motility may result in unpredictable drug absorption. Therefore, in the symptomatic patient, it may be preferable to convert these medications to the parenteral route. A patient who has required systemic steroid therapy within the previous 4 weeks should receive intravenous hydrocor-

Table 3.1 *Intrapartum management of asthma*

ADMISSION ASSESSMENT

History and physical examination

Peak expiratory flow rate (PEFR) measurement

Oxygenation status (pulse oximetry, arterial blood gas)

CONTROLLED ASTHMA

Definition

PEFR ≥ 80% baseline

Asymptomatic

Continue routine antenatal asthma medications

Administer IV hydrocortisone (100 mg q8h) until 24 hr postpartum if patient was treated with steroids during past 4 wk

Analgesia

Avoid morphine and meperidine

Consider fentanyl

Consider epidural anesthesia

EXACERBATION OF ASTHMA

Definition

PEFR < 80% baseline

Symptomatic: wheezes, cough, dyspnea, chest tightness

Treatment

Inhaled, subcutaneous or intravenous beta-2 agonist

Intravenous corticosteroids (hydrocortisone, 4-mg/kg bolus, then 3 mg/kg every 4–6 hr)

Continuous pulse oximetry

Oxygen to maintain saturation > 95%

Serial PEFR assessment

Analgesia (as in controlled asthma)

Continuous fetal monitoring

tisone (100 mg every 8 hours) throughout labor and for 24 hours postpartum to prevent adrenal insufficiency. There are no laboratory studies specifically required in the pregnant asthmatic with the exception of measurement of the baseline theophylline level if this has been a part of the antepartum medication regimen. Routine arterial blood gas analysis is not required in the clinically stable patient.

Evidence for an acute exacerbation of asthma during labor includes a peak flow rate less than 80% of baseline, shortness of breath, or wheezing. Underlying etiologies such as pulmonary edema, infection, or cardiac failure should always be investigated. Previously, the mainstay of acute treatment focused on the use of intravenous theophylline preparations (6). Although this approach has fallen into disfavor, the following are generally used dosage parameters: a loading dose of aminophylline (5 mg/kg of ideal body weight over 30 minutes) is followed by a maintenance infusion (0.8 mg/kg/hr). Serum levels are measured 1 to 2 hours after initiation of therapy. The infusion rate can be adjusted to maintain a therapeutic level of 10 to 20 µg/mL. Common side effects include gastrointestinal intolerance, tachycardia, and palpitations. Patients taking erythromycin should be observed for theophylline toxicity due to the decreased clearance of the latter.

More recently, aggressive treatment with beta-2 agonists and intravenous steroids are recommended as first-line agents (7). Beta-2 agonists can be administered in an aerosolized fashion to minimize systemic absorption. Nebulized albuterol (Ventolin) is administered by preparing 2.5–5.0 mg (0.5–1.0 mL of a 0.5% inhalation solution) in 2.5 mL of sterile saline solution. Alternatively, the beta-2 agonists may be given subcutaneously or intravenously (e.g., terbutaline, 0.25 mg). Side effects of this class of agents include tachycardia and hypotension; the fetus should be continuously monitored. Although the beta agonists have been used to prevent preterm delivery, there are no data to suggest that these agents interfere with the overall course of labor and delivery at term in the asthmatic. Steroids can likewise be administered via an inhaled or intravenous route. Most often, in the acute setting, intravenous hydrocortisone is given as a bolus dose (4 mg/kg) followed by 3 mg/kg every 4 to 6 hours. Side effects of short-term steroid therapy are unusual, although the long-term use of these agents has the potential for a multitude of adverse effects.

In the symptomatic patient, serial arterial blood gas determinations may be required depending on the initial blood gas result. Placement of a radial arterial line is helpful when it is apparent that repeated sampling will be necessary to manage maternal oxygenation. In the patient with an oxygen saturation greater than 95%, pulse oximetry can be used as a noninvasive method of estimating oxygenation. Intubation and mechanical ventilation become necessary when the patient demonstrates signs of respiratory failure (Table 3.2) (8). Although threshold parameters are offered as guidelines, the patient's clinical status should be taken into consideration with the understanding that it is preferable to intubate a patient in a controlled setting, prior to respiratory failure. Vaginal delivery remains the preferred method of delivery even with severe exacerbation because of the significantly increased pulmonary risks associated with

Table 3.2 *General guidelines for initiating mechanical ventilation in patients with asthma*

Parameter	Threshold values
P_{O_2}	< 70 mm Hg (with $F_{I}O_2$ 0.4 by mask)
	< 300 mm Hg (with $F_{I}O_2$ 1.0)
P_{CO_2}	> 35 mm Hg
Respiratory rate	> 35 breaths/min
PEFR	≤ 25% baseline

PEFR—peak expiratory flow rate; $F_{I}O_2$—fraction of inspired oxygen.

cesarean delivery. Supine positioning during the labor and delivery process should be avoided.

Since the anxiety and hyperventilation associated with labor and delivery may exacerbate asthma, adequate analgesia should be provided. Intravenous morphine and meperidine have been associated with histamine release and bronchospasm (9). Therefore, fentanyl is considered by some to be the preferred intravenous agent. Conduction anesthesia has the advantage of providing excellent pain relief with minimal respiratory depression. A high thoracic block, however, should be avoided since unopposed parasympathetic tone may cause bronchoconstriction. General anesthesia also carries an increased risk of bronchospasm. When possible, the patient should receive adequate preoperative preparation, including hydration and prophylactic beta-2-agonist inhaler treatment. Induction of anesthesia with ketamine has some advantage, in that this agent is a bronchodilator and does not cause histamine release.

In the event of postpartum hemorrhage due to uterine atony, intravenous oxytocin remains the therapy of choice. Methylergonovine maleate (Methergine) (0.2 mg given intramuscularly) should be employed as second-line therapy for uterine atony unresponsive to oxytocin since 15-methylprostaglandin $F_{2\alpha}$ (250 µg given intramuscularly) has been associated with bronchospasm and oxygen desaturation (4). If prostaglandins must be used in a patient with mild to moderate asthma, premedication with steroids (e.g., intravenous hydrocortisone, 100 mg) and diphenhydramine (50 mg given intravenously) should be instituted.

Following delivery, the patient should receive humidifed oxygen, aggressive incentive spirometry, and beta-2-agonist aerosol treatments. This is particularly true in the patient who has undergone cesarean delivery with resultant postoperative atelectasis. Chest physiotherapy can be instituted as deemed necessary. The patient's antepartum medication regimen and stress steroids (if required) should be continued into the postpartum period. As soon as the patient is able to tolerate oral intake, intravenous agents may be converted to their oral counterparts.

PULMONARY EMBOLISM

Pulmonary embolism (PE) should be considered in the differential diagnosis of any patient experiencing acute onset of shortness of breath. Although the highest-risk period is postpartum, venous thrombosis and embolism can occur at any time in pregnancy. The presenting signs of tachypnea and dyspnea occur in 90 and 80%, respectively, of patients with a pulmonary embolism (10).

Additional signs and symptoms include pleuritic chest pain, apprehension, cough, diaphoresis, atelectatic rales, hemoptysis, fever, cyanosis, and heart sound changes. Signs of right-sided heart failure are associated when a massive embolus occludes more than 50% of the pulmonary circulation.

The diagnosis of PE is based on a high degree of clinical suspicion. An arterial blood gas with a partial pressure of oxygen (PO_2) less than 85 mm Hg is very suggestive, although 14% of patients with angiographically proved PE have a PO_2 above 85 mm Hg (11). The chest radiograph may appear normal in 30% of patients (12), but its primary role is in excluding other chest pathology and aiding in lung scan interpretation. The electrocardiogram most commonly shows sinus tachycardia. Right axis shift with the S1 Q3 T3 pattern and nonspecific T-wave changes occur only with massive embolism. With the exception of an arterial blood gas analysis, other laboratory studies are not helpful in the diagnosis of PE. The ventilation-perfusion scan has a positive predictive value of 90% whether or not it is combined with noninvasive studies for deep venous thrombosis (13). Pulmonary arteriography is the definitive procedure for the diagnosis of PE when the lung scan findings are indeterminate or indicate moderate probability, or do not correlate with a high clinical suspicion.

When a PE is suspected, multiple diagnostic and therapeutic actions may be simultaneously required. Oxygen should be administered to maintain a PO_2 above 60 mm Hg to ensure adequate fetal oxygenation. Continuous fetal heart rate monitoring should be instituted as soon as possible. Anticoagulation should begin immediately and prior to further diagnostic testing. If there is no evidence of a PE following the evaluation, heparin may then be discontinued. The initial intravenous heparin bolus is administered as 70 to 100 U/kg (5000–10,000 total units) followed by a maintenance infusion at a rate of 15 to 20 U/kg/hour (approximately 1000 U/hr). Blood should be drawn prior to administration of the heparin bolus to establish a baseline value of the activated partial thromboplastin time (aPTT). The maintenance infusion of heparin can be adjusted to achieve an aPTT 2.0 to 2.5 times above the patient's baseline value. Alternatively, heparin levels may allow more accurate administration of this anticoagulant; the therapeutic level ranges from 0.2 to 0.4 unit/mL. This test, however, may not be available in many institutions. Intrapartum management of the anticoagulated patient is discussed further in a subsequent chapter.

▦ PULMONARY EDEMA

Pulmonary edema can be broadly classified as cardiogenic or noncardiogenic. Cardiogenic edema results from left ventricular failure, while noncardiogenic edema is caused by pulmonary endothelial damage and increased capillary permeability. Although cardiogenic and noncardiogenic pulmonary edema have two distinct pathophysiologies, they share the common final pathway of increased interstitial and intra-alveolar fluid. Inciting factors of pulmonary edema are listed Table 3.3.

Regardless of the etiology, the goals of treatment include: 1) adequate maternal oxygenation, 2) removal of excess fluid, and 3) treatment of the inciting cause. Oxygen therapy and elevation of the head of the

Table 3.3 *Inciting factors of pulmonary edema*

Beta-mimetic tocolytics

Iatrogenic fluid overload

Severe preeclampsia

Sepsis

Aspiration pneumonia

Blood transfusion

Disseminated intravascular coagulopathy

Cardiac failure

Amniotic fluid embolus

patient's bed are basic steps in managing patients with pulmonary edema. The initial room air arterial blood gas result will guide oxygen therapy; the PO_2 should be maintained above 60 mm Hg to ensure adequate fetal oxygenation. Pulse oximetry with saturations of more than 95% may be utilized when the patient is not severely hypoxic. It should be noted that oximetry data are limited by the nature of the oxygen dissociation curve, in that a patient with a saturation of 95% may have a PO_2 as low as 70 mm Hg.

Diuresis with furosemide is the mainstay of treatment; the initial dose is 20 to 40 mg as an intravenous bolus. If no response is observed within 1 hour, the dose may be doubled. Morphine sulfate will cause pulmonary venous dilatation, relieve maternal anxiety, and decrease the work of breathing. An initial intravenous dose of 3 to 5 mg can be repeated every 15 minutes to a maximum of 15 mg in a 3- to 4-hour period. Care should be taken to avoid excessive narcotic dosing, as the resultant respiratory depression may further compromise the borderline patient. Determination and treatment of the precipitating condition should begin immediately. As the patient improves, surveillance of urinary output, serum electrolyte levels, pulse oximetry, and lung examination should continue.

When the patient's clinical condition fails to improve with this approach, invasive monitoring should be considered to accurately determine the patient's hemodynamic status. Further therapy is aimed at reducing the pulmonary capillary wedge pressure while improving cardiac output. Mechanical ventilation should not be delayed in the patient who continues to show signs of respiratory compromise (see Table 3.2).

Although many conditions associated with pulmonary edema (e.g., preeclampsia) mandate delivery of the fetus in a timely fashion, initial attempts at maternal stabilization should reduce the risk of fetal distress. Vaginal delivery is the preferred route of delivery, and cesarean section should be reserved for standard obstetric indications. It should be anticipated that the patient may experience an exacerbation of pulmonary edema following delivery secondary to the physiologic redistribution of intravascular volume. Therefore careful surveillance of intake and output must be continued into the postpartum period.

■ REFERENCES

1. Weinstein AM, Dubin BD, Podleski WK, Spector SL, Raff RS. Asthma and pregnancy. JAMA 1979;241:1161–65.

2. Hernandez E, Angell CS, Johnson JWG. Asthma in pregnancy: current concepts. Obstet Gynecol 1980;55:739–43.

3. Schaefer G, Silverman F. Pregnancy complicated by asthma. Am J Obstet Gynecol 1961;82:182–91.

4. Hankins GD, Berryman GK, Scott RT, Hood D. Maternal arterial desaturation with 15-methyl prostaglandin F_2 alpha for uterine atony. Obstet Gynecol 1988;72:367–70.

5. National Heart, Lung, and Blood Institute. Management of asthma during pregnancy. National Institutes of Health Publication No. 93-3279A. Bethesda, MD: National Institutes of Health, October 1992:5.

6. Barnes PJ. A new approach to the treatment of asthma. N Engl J Med 1989;321:1517–25.

7. Siege D, Sheppard D, Gelb A, et al. Aminophylline increases the toxicity but not the efficacy of an inhaled beta-adrenergic agonist in the treatment of acute exacerbations of asthma. Am Rev Respir Dis 1985;132:283.

8. Hankins GDV. Acute pulmonary injury and respiratory failure during pregnancy. In: Clark SL, Cotton DB, Hankins GDV, Phelan JP, eds. Critical care obstetrics. 2nd ed. Cambridge: Blackwell Scientific Publications, 1987:357.

9. Hermens JM, Ebertz JM, Hanifin JM, Hirshman CA. Comparison of histamine release in human skin mast cells induced by morphine, fentanyl, and oxymorphone. Anesthesiology 1985;62:124–29.

10. Laros RK, Alger LS. Thromboembolism and pregnancy. Clin Obstet Gynecol 1979;22:871–88.

11. Robin ED. Overdiagnosis and overtreatment of pulmonary embolism: the emperor may have no clothes. Ann Intern Med 1977;87:775–781.

12. Rosenow EC III, Osmundson PJ, Brown ML. Pulmonary embolism. Mayo Clin Proc 1981;56:161–178.

13. Alderson PO. Scintigraphic evaluation of pulmonary embolism. Eur J Nucl Med 1987;13:S6–S10.

Liver Disease

▼   ▼   ▼   ▼   ▼

■ ACUTE FATTY LIVER OF PREGNANCY

Acute fatty liver of pregnancy (AFLP) typically occurs in the third trimester and is characterized by microvesicular fatty liver infiltration. Hepatic and renal failure, hypoglycemia, metabolic acidosis, coagulopathy, and encephalopathy may rapidly develop. AFLP is frequently associated with primiparity, twin gestation, and preeclampsia. Maternal and neonatal survival rates have improved in recent times due to an increased awareness and aggressive treatment of the disease. Early recognition and delivery combined with supportive care optimize pregnancy outcome.

The mean gestational age at presentation is 36 weeks. Symptoms may include nausea, vomiting, anorexia, malaise, and abdominal pain. The patient often appears ill and jaundiced. Physical examination may reveal hypertension, a small to normal-sized liver, edema, ascites, spider hemangiomas, and palmar erythema. Neurologic function may be intact or range from confusion to obtundation, with asterixis often present.

AFLP is most frequently confused with HELLP (hemolysis, elevated liver enzymes, and low platelets) syndrome (Table 4.1). The differential diagnosis also includes thrombotic thrombocytopenic purpura (TTP),

Table 4.1 *Laboratory differentiation of AFLP and HELLP syndrome**

	AFLP	HELLP
Hematologic		
Platelet count	Low or normal	Low
Fibrinogen	Low	Normal to increased
Prothrombin time (PT)	Prolonged	Normal
Partial thromboplastin time (PTT)	Prolonged	Normal
Serum chemistries		
Glucose	Low	Normal
Uric acid	High	High
Creatinine	High	High
Ammonia	High	Normal

*Reprinted by permission from Barton JR, Sibai BM. Care of the pregnancy complicated by HELLP syndrome. Obstet Gynecol Clin North Am 1991;18:165–179.

hemolytic-uremic syndrome (HUS), acute viral hepatitis, and cholestasis of pregnancy (see Table 1.6). Thus a variety of laboratory studies may be required to establish the diagnosis. The laboratory evaluation of a patient with suspected AFLP includes a complete blood cell count with differential and platelet count; prothrombin time (PT); partial thromboplastin time (PTT); measurements of fibrinogen, serum electrolytes, blood urea nitrogen (BUN) and creatinine, alanine aminotransferase (ALT), aspartate aminotransferase (AST), bilirubin, ammonia, amylase, and uric acid levels; and urinalysis. Hepatitis profiles will exclude it as the etiology of liver disease. Ultrasonography, computed tomography, and magnetic resonance imaging have been used in an attempt to diagnose AFLP, but normal findings on these studies are not exclusionary (1,2). The definitive diagnosis is based on liver histology with special staining for fat such as with oil red O. Percutaneous liver biopsy, however, is unnecessary if clinical and laboratory evidence supports the diagnosis.

Once AFLP is suspected, it is important that critical care support be immediately available in the event of acute liver failure. Vital signs should be monitored every 1 to 2 hours. Pulse oximetry allows assessment of pulmonary status and early detection of respiratory compromise. Given the increased risk of fetal compromise, fetal heart rate monitoring should be instituted on admission. Since acute renal failure commonly accompanies hepatic failure, a urethral catheter should be placed. Urine output and fluid intake must be accurately recorded. Serial monitoring of laboratory values is essential. To monitor for hypoglycemia, blood glucose concentration should be measured every 1 to 2 hours with a bedside glucometer. As a general rule, electrolyte and coagulation studies should be performed every 4 to 6 hours. Because some authorities have suggested that preeclampsia may coexist with AFLP (3,4), treatment with magnesium sulfate should be instituted if there is any suspicion of this complicating factor. Hypertension may require treatment with hydralazine or other anti-hypertensive agents.

Aggressive treatment of the complications of AFLP is required. Electrolyte and metabolic derangements should be corrected. Hypoglycemia can be treated with a 5 to 20% dextrose infusion to maintain the blood glucose concentration above 60 mg/dL. Due to the increased risk of hemorrhagic complications, transfusion with packed red blood cells should be considered when the hemoglobin falls below 8 gm/dL. Fresh frozen plasma and platelets are administered to correct coagulopathy. Hepatic failure and encephalopathy are treated with sodium restriction and oral or rectal lactulose. Mechanical ventilation is required when there is pulmonary failure. Additional complications that may require treatment include pancreatitis, gastrointestinal bleeding, acute renal failure, pulmonary embolism, and transient diabetes insipidus (> 3 liters of urine/day with urine osmolality < 200 mOsm and continuous thirst).

Plans for prompt delivery of the fetus should be instituted as soon as attempts have been made to stabilize the maternal condition. There is no evidence, however, that cesarean section affords a better outcome in the absence of fetal distress. Thus, vaginal delivery may be attempted, but a specific time period should be determined for establishment of active labor. Conduction anesthesia is preferred in the absence of coagulation abnormalities. Because the metabolism of many anesthetic agents is via the liver, general anesthesia is associated with increased risks in the presence of hepatic dysfunction. Postpartum, intensive surveillance must be continued as complications of the disease may still occur in the initial hours following delivery. The natural course of AFLP is one of improvement over the 2 to 3 days following delivery.

▓ LIVER HEMATOMA AND RUPTURE

Although spontaneous liver rupture during pregnancy is uncommon, it carries a maternal mortality rate of 60%. It is most frequently associated with severe preeclampsia/eclampsia. Henny et al (5) described two phases of subcapsular hematoma and rupture. A prodromal phase consists of headache, nausea, and vomiting with progression to severe right-upper-quadrant (RUQ) pain and signs of hypertension. The second phase is the actual rupture of the subcapsular hematoma. Pain may increase in intensity and radiate to the right shoulder due to diaphragmatic irritation by blood. Rapid deterioration of the patient with hypotension, shock, and fetal distress may ensue. The triad of preeclampsia, RUQ pain, and shock should raise the suspicion of a liver rupture. The clinical presentation, however, can be extremely variable and often hinders the diagnosis.

Frequent monitoring of vital signs, urine output, and hematocrit should be performed in any patient suspected of having a liver hematoma or rupture. A subcapsular hematoma can be diagnosed using computed tomography, ultrasonography, magnetic resonance imaging, or radionuclide scanning. Recently, conservative management of subcapsular hematomas was suggested, owing to the increased risks associated with surgical evacuation (6–8). Long-term, serial ultrasonography is recommended until resolution of the hematoma is documented. Delivery, however, should be effected to minimize perinatal and maternal mortality.

A patient who is hemodynamically unstable should be taken for emergent laparotomy without delay. While preparations for delivery are being made, venous access with large-bore catheters should be secured and fluid resuscitation initiated. Preoperative consultation with a general or vascular surgeon for immediate intraoperative assistance may be beneficial. A type and crossmatch for 6 units of packed red blood cells should be available in the blood bank. The blood bank should be notified of the potential need for massive transfusion of packed cells as well as platelets and fresh frozen plasma. A midline vertical incision will allow optimal access to the liver. Packing of the RUQ on entering the abdomen can be performed to tamponade the bleeding. Delivery of a viable fetus should occur as quickly as possible so that attention can be focused on the site of hemorrhage. Even in the event of a fetal demise, emptying of the uterus may be necessary to provide adequate exposure of the upper abdomen.

Various techniques for repair of a liver laceration have been described (9). Evacuation of the hematoma is followed by mechanical compression of the area. Suturing, topical coagulants, omental pedicles, hepatic artery ligation, arterial embolization, and lobectomy have all been performed. The hepatic bed is usually drained with a Penrose or sump drain through a separate stab incision. When all other measures have failed, packing of the hepatic bed and closure of the abdomen have been used.

Postoperatively, invasive hemodynamic monitoring may be required to accurately assess the patient's volume status. When massive transfusions of blood products have been given, the patient is at risk of developing adult respiratory distress syndrome. Ongoing anemia and coagulopathy may require continued transfusion and replacement with blood products during the initial 24 to 48 hours following surgery.

◼ LIVER CIRRHOSIS

Liver cirrhosis is associated with a variety of infectious, metabolic, hereditary, and drug-related disorders. The characteristic pathologic feature is chronic parenchymal injury with extensive fibrosis and regenerative nodules. It is an entity associated with a wide spectrum of clinical manifestations. Jaundice, edema, coagulopathy, and metabolic aberrations may result from loss of functioning hepatocytes. The fibrosis and abnormal vasculature lead to portal hypertension and its associated complications of splenomegaly and esophageal varices. Encephalopathy and ascites are due to the combination of hepatocellular insufficiency and portal hypertension.

Pregnancy is uncommon in women with cirrhosis, and limited information is available. Cirrhotic patients without jaundice or impaired liver function often have successful term pregnancies. Maternal prognosis in the presence of cirrhosis depends on the degree of hepatic dysfunction more than the etiology of the disease (10). Bleeding from esophageal varices remains the most significant maternal risk during pregnancy. The fetus is at an increased risk of stillbirth and neonatal death.

Any patient with liver cirrhosis should undergo delivery where intensive care facilities are immediately available. Laboratory values obtained at the onset of labor should include hemoglobin, hematocrit, platelet count, AST, ALT, PT, PTT, fibrinogen, and a blood type and screen. If there is evidence of a coagulopathy, the need for packed red blood cells, fresh frozen plasma or cryoprecipitate, and platelets must be anticipated.

Vaginal delivery may be allowed, but a shortened second stage of labor should be considered to prevent the increased portal pressure associated with straining. Cesarean section is reserved for standard obstetric indications. Abdominal delivery may be complicated by an extensive collateral circulation or adhesive disease following portocaval shunt placement. Postpartum hemorrhage has been known to occur more frequently in patients who have undergone portocaval shunting (10). Intrapartum analgesia is optimally provided with conduction anesthesia. Because of diminished liver function, intravenous analgesics as well as anesthetic agents have increased serum half-lives, and if they are utilized, dosing should be adjusted accordingly.

Postpartum, the patient must be closely observed for signs of decompensation. Bleeding from esophageal varices continues to be the most significant risk. Hepatic encephalopathy can be precipitated during the intrapartum and postpartum periods by a variety of factors including blood loss, hypotension, hypoglycemia, infection, thiazide diuretics, and anesthetic agents. Thus, liver function tests and coagulation studies should be performed serially to monitor for increasing hepatic dysfunction following delivery.

■ HEPATITIS

Viral hepatitis is the most common cause of jaundice in pregnancy. The etiology of hepatitis includes hepatitis A, B, C, D, and E viruses as well as cytomegalovirus and Epstein-Barr, herpes simplex, and varicella-zoster viruses. Diagnosis is based on the various serologic markers associated with each virus. Hepatitis B virus has been reported to be the most common etiologic agent in pregnancy. Patients with acute hepatitis during the third trimester are at risk for premature delivery as well as vertical transmission to the fetus. Few data are available regarding the intrapartum management of many of the above-mentioned viral pathogens; therefore the remainder of this discussion focuses on hepatitis A, B, and C viruses.

Hepatitis A Virus

Hepatitis A virus is transmitted via the fecal-oral route with an incubation period of 15 to 50 days. Symptoms of disease include fatigue, anorexia, fever, weakness, arthralgias, and headache, followed by jaundice, dark urine, and light stools. Liver enlargement and tenderness may be present on physical examination. IgM antibody to hepatitis A virus is diagnostic of acute infection. When patients with active hepatitis A present in labor, infectious disease precautions should be followed as the virus is excreted in the stool during the acute phase. In addition to standard admission laboratory studies, the following parameters should be measured: AST, ALT, direct and indirect bilirubin, PT, PTT, fibrinogen, and platelet count. If the results of the coagulation studies are abnormal, fresh frozen plasma should be available. If the patient has signs of active bleeding or a platelet count of less than 50,000/mm (3) with plans for operative delivery, 10 units of platelets should be administered. Although there is no evidence of vertical transmission of the hepatitis A virus to the fetus, Klion has recommend immune serum immunoglobulin administration to the neonate after delivery because of the risk of transmission from infected maternal stool (11).

Hepatitis B Virus

The frequencies of acute and chronic hepatitis B in pregnancy are 1 to 2 per 1000 and 10 to 15 per 1000, respectively (12). Patients at high risk for hepatitis B infection include health care workers, intravenous drug abusers, sexual partners of bisexual men, those with multiple sexual partners, patients from endemic areas (Asia, Pacific Islands, Haiti, sub-Sahara Africa), patients with a history of transfusions, and household contacts of patients with acute or chronic hepatitis B infection. Because risk factors alone do not identify an adequate number of infected women, current recommendations are to employ universal screening in pregnancy.

The diagnosis of hepatitis B infection is based on the identification of specific antigen and antibody serologic markers (Figure 4.1). Persistence of hepatitis surface antigenemia for longer than 6 months implies chronic infection (carrier state). Patients infected with hepatitis B in the first and second trimesters have a less than 10% risk

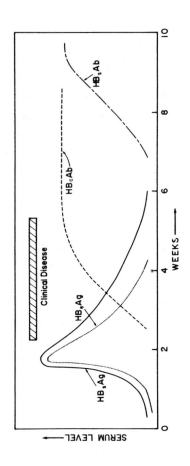

Fig. 4.1 *Immunologic characteristics of hepatitis B. (Reprinted by permission from Fallon HJ. Liver diseases. In: Burrow GN, Ferris TF, eds. Medical complications during pregnancy. 3rd ed. Philadelphia: WB Saunders Company, 1988:331.)*

of vertical transmission. Conversely, those acutely infected in the third trimester have a 65% risk of transmission. Of particular importance is that the risk of perinatal transmission of hepatitis B in the chronic carrier can be directly correlated to the presence of hepatitis B e antigen (HBeAg). The perinatal transmission risk is 75 to 90% with a positive HBeAg finding while the risk is 5% when the HBeAg finding is negative. Neonates contracting hepatitis B infection at delivery have an approximately 90% chance of developing chronic hepatitis B surface antigen (HBsAg) carriage and subsequent liver disease such as cirrhosis and hepatoma formation.

When the patient with acute hepatitis B infection presents at term, the clinical picture may be complicated and confused with other intrapartum conditions (see Table 1.6). Among the symptoms seen with acute infection are nausea, malaise, fatigue, photophobia, arthralgias, and headaches. These symptoms are usually seen 1 to 2 weeks prior to the onset of jaundice (seen when bilirubin > 2.5 mg/dL). Hepatic enzymes (ALT and AST) are elevated along with the serum bilirubin. Symptomatic support with hydration and antiemetics are appropriate maternal management interventions. The risk of perinatal transmission of hepatitis B virus is specifically related to fetal contact with maternal blood and vaginal secretions at delivery. Fetal scalp electrodes and blood sampling should be avoided if possible. Cesarean delivery should be reserved for obstetric indications. The nursery staff should be aware of the patient's status so they can administer hepatitis B immune globulin (HBIG) to the newborn (0.5 mL immediately after birth, followed by the series of hepatits B vaccines) (13).

Hepatitis C Virus

Hepatitis C virus (HCV), previously referred to as non-A, non-B hepatitis, is a common cause of both acute and chronic liver disease (14). Hepatitis C accounts for approximately 5% of all reported cases of infectious hepatitis. Up to 50% of acute hepatits C infections result in progression to chronic liver disease. HCV is the major etiologic agent for transfusion-related hepatitis. Risk factors for infection are epidemiologically similar to those associated with the hepatitis B virus, and a significant proportion of infected individuals escape detection when screening protocols are based on risk factors alone (15). Rates of HCV antibody seropositivity in pregnancy range from 2.3 to 4.5% (16). Vertical transmission to the newborn occurs in less than 5% of cases, although this rate significantly increases in parturients with high viral titers, HCV-RNA–positive cord blood, and human immunodeficiency virus (HIV) coinfection (14,16–18). Short- and long-term consequences of perinatal vertical transmission have yet to be adequately defined. Intrapartum management for HCV-infected gravidas should be similar to that described for hepatitis B infection. At present, routine serologic screening is not advocated as a cost-effective measure, in particular because no neonatal HCV-specific prophylaxis has been recommended.

■ REFERENCES

1. Mabie WC, Dacus JV, Sibai BM, Morretti ML, Gold RE. Computed tomography in acute fatty liver of pregnancy. Am J Obstet Gynecol 1988;158:142–385.

2. Campillo B, Bernuau J, Witz MO, et al. Ultrasonography in acute fatty liver of pregnancy. Ann Intern Med 1986; 105:383–384.

3. Burroughs AK, Seong NH, Dojcinar DM, et al. Idiopathic acute fatty liver of pregnancy in 12 patients. Q J Med 1982; 204:481.

4. Riely CA, Latham PS, Romero R, et al. Acute fatty liver of pregnancy. A reassessment based on observations in nine patients. Ann Intern Med 1987;106:703.

5. Henny CP, Lim AE, Brummelkamp WH, Buller HR, Ten Cate JW. A review of the importance of acute multidisciplinary treatment following spontaneous rupture of the liver capsule during pregnancy. Surg Gynecol Obstet 1983; 156:593–598.

6. Lavery JP, Berg J. Subcapsular hematoma of the liver during pregnancy. South Med J 1989;82:1568–1570.

7. Manas KJ, Welsh JD, Rankin RA, et al. Hepatic hemorrhage without rupture in preeclampsia. N Engl J Med 1985;312:424–425.

8. Goodlin RC, Anderson JC, Hodgson PE. Conservative treatment of liver hematoma in the postpartum period. A report of two cases. J Reprod Med 1985;80:368–370.

9. Herbert WNP, Brenner WE. Improving survival with liver rupture complicating pregnancy. Am J Obstet Gynecol 1982;142:530–534.

10. Cheng YS. Pregnancy in liver cirrhosis and/or portal hypertension. Am J Obstet Gynecol 1977;128:812–822.

11. Klion FM. Liver in normal pregnancy. In: Cherry SH, Merkatz IR, eds. Complications of pregnancy: medical, surgical, gynecologic, psychosocial, and perinatal. 4th ed. Baltimore: Williams & Wilkins, 1991:800.

12. Simms J, Duff P. Viral hepatitis in pregnancy. Semin Perinatol 1993;17:384–393.

13. Paz I, Seidman DS, Mashiach S, Stevenson DK. Maternal

transmission of human immunodeficiency virus-1. Obstet Gynecol Surv 1994;49:577–584.

14. Lynch-Salamon D, Coombs CA. Hepatitis C in obstetrics and gynecology. Obstet Gynecol 1992;79:621–629.

15. Reinus JF, Leikin EL, Alter HJ, et al. Failure to detect vertical transmission of hepatitis C virus. Ann Intern Med 1992;117:881–886.

16. Silverman NS, Jenkin BK, Wu C, et al. Hepatitis C virus in pregnancy: seroprevalence and risk factors for infection. Am J Obstet Gynecol 1993;169:583–587.

17. Lin HH, Kao JH, Hsu H, et al. Possible role of high titer maternal viremia in perinatal transmission of hepatitis C virus. J Infect Dis 1994;169:638–641.

18. Ohto H, Terazawa S, Sasaki N, et al. Transmission of hepatitis C virus from mothers to infants. N Engl J Med 1994; 330:744–750.

Renal Disease

▼   ▼   ▼   ▼   ▼

▓ OLIGURIA AND ACUTE RENAL FAILURE

Acute renal failure occurs in less than 1% of pregnancies. Broadly defined, this condition is characterized by a rapid deterioration in renal function with resultant accumulation of nitrogenous products in the blood. The normal creatinine concentration during pregnancy of 0.5 to 0.7 mg/dL and mean blood urea nitrogen concentration of 9 mg/dL are due to the 50% increase in glomerular filtration rate. As renal function is compromised, the clearance of creatinine and urea decreases, and azotemia (an increase in serum urea and creatinine levels) develops. Thus, a serum creatinine level higher than 1 mg/dL should be considered abnormal in a pregnant woman.

The term *acute renal failure* has generated a great deal of confusion in that some clinicians limit this diagnosis to intrinsic renal disease, while others include prerenal azotemia, obstructive uropathy, and even oliguria within this definition. Additional confusion relates to the fact that these latter conditions can eventually lead to intrinsic renal damage, and therefore may truly be etiologic depending on the time course. Lastly, there is a subset of patients in whom renal failure is present in the absence of oliguria (1).

The most common reason a patient in labor will be

evaluated for renal failure is oliguria. Oliguria is strictly defined as a urine output of less than 400 mL/24 hours, but a urinary output of less than 30 mL/hour for 2 consecutive hours is often considered clinical evidence of oliguria. Three categories are used to classify the etiology of oliguria (Table 5.1). Nonrenal prerenal azotemia is characterized by a decrease in intravascular volume and renal perfusion with a resultant increase in salt and water retention by the kidney. Acute tubular necrosis secondary to ischemia and nephrotoxicity accounts for the majority of intrinsic renal disease causing oliguria. Obstruction is the least common cause of oliguria and renal failure.

Patients may initially be without clinical signs or symptoms except for increasing serum urea nitrogen and creatinine levels. However, if renal function has begun to deteriorate significantly prior to the diagnosis of acute renal failure, the patient may have signs and symptoms attributable to uremia, including edema, hypertension, nausea, vomiting, bleeding, or changes in mental status.

Whenever decreased urine output is suspected, a urethral catheter should be placed. Urine and serum electrolyte measurements may be helpful in determining the etiology of the oliguria (Table 5.2) (2). However, as previously discussed, these parameters have not been shown to be valid when the patient has oliguria associated with preeclampsia (3). Diuretic administration will also alter the usefulness of these urinary diagnostic indices. If urine electrolyte values indicate prerenal azotemia, initial management is directed at replacement of intravascular volume. Administration of 500 to 1000 mL of normal saline solution followed by maintenance fluid at 150 to 200 mL/hour is commonly employed in

Table 5.1 *Etiology of oliguria*

Nonrenal/Prerenal causes

Volume depletion

Hemorrhage

Dehydration

Sepsis

Cardiac failure

Intrinsic renal disease

Acute tubular necrosis

Ischemia

Toxic

Glomerular disease

Interstitial nephritis

Vascular disease

Malignant hypertension

Renal artery obstruction

Obstructive/postrenal

Ureteral obstruction

Causes unique to pregnancy

Preeclampsia-eclampsia

HELLP syndrome

Pelvic hematoma

Amniotic fluid embolism

Acute fatty liver of pregnancy

Polyhydramnios

Table 5.2 *Urinary indices in acute renal failure*

	Prerenal azotemia	*Acute tubular necrosis*	*Obstructive uropathy*
Specific gravity	> 1.020	< 1.010	
Urine osmolality (mOsm/kg H_2O)	> 350	< 400	< 400
Urine sodium (mEq/L)	< 20	> 40	> 30
Urine/plasma creatinine	> 40	< 20	< 20
Fractional excretion of sodium (FE_{Na})*	< 1	> 1	> 1

*$FE_{Na} = \dfrac{\text{urine}_{Na}/\text{serum}_{Na}}{\text{urine}_{Cr}/\text{serum}_{Cr}} \times 100.$

this setting. Fluid replacement may be continued as deemed necessary, with care not to overload the patient. Chest auscultation should be performed frequently to detect early signs of pulmonary edema.

If urine output does not improve following intravenous fluid administration, central hemodynamic monitoring with a pulmonary artery catheter is indicated. Volume replacement may then continue when the hemodynamic parameters indicate a decreased intravascular volume. If the patient remains oliguric in spite of an optimized volume status or intrinsic renal disease is suspected, furosemide (1.5–6.0 mg/kg every 2–4 hours) is an appropriate therapeutic intervention. Renal dose dopamine (1.5–5.0 µg/kg/min) has also been used to increase renal perfusion (4). A bedside renal ultrasound can be attempted to rule out renal obstruction, although this study will be of limited usefulness in the laboring gravida. The remainder of the intrapartum management plan is limited to a careful balancing of intake and output, surveillance of electrolyte values, and careful monitoring of medications that are excreted by the renal system (Table 5.3). Dialysis and nutritional considerations should await the postpartum period, with the anticipation that in most patients acute renal failure will be self-limited. This is, of course, assuming that the underlying etiology has been recognized and the duration of renal insult was short.

THE TRANSPLANT PATIENT

An increasing number of women who have undergone renal transplantation are now attempting pregnancy; of

Table 5.3 *Medications commonly used in pregnancy with significant renal excretion*

Acyclovir
Aminoglycosides
Ampicillin
Aztreonam
Cefazolin
Cimetidine
Ibuprofen
Magnesium sulfate
Phenytoin
Ranitidine

pregnancies that continue beyond the first trimester, 90% have a successful outcome (5,6). The major maternal risks include infection, hypertension, preeclampsia, worsening renal function, and graft rejection. Preeclampsia has been noted to develop in approximately 30% of transplant patients (7). The most important predictors of pregnancy outcome include the preconception serum creatinine level, presence or absence of hypertension, immunosuppressive regimen, and time since transplantation. It is also important to be mindful of the underlying medical condition that necessitated the transplantation. The fetus is at an increased risk of premature delivery, intrauterine growth restriction, and infection.

On admission to the labor and delivery unit, serum blood urea nitrogen (BUN), creatinine, and cyclosporine levels (as indicated) should be measured. If the patient has had adequate renal function, serum electrolyte values are expected to be within normal limits. The patient's hepatitis B virus and human immunodeficiency virus (HIV) status should be known as this group of patients frequently have been exposed to multiple blood products.

Vital signs should be closely monitored because a hypertensive crisis can occur very rapidly in patients with renal disease. This hypertension should be aggressively treated as outlined previously for the nontransplant patient (see Table 1.5). The signs of preeclampsia, however, are often difficult to distinguish from the underlying hypertension, proteinuria, and elevated uric acid level frequently associated with renal disease. Acute tissue rejection and immunosuppressive drug toxicity can further confuse the clinical picture. Approximately 40% of gravidas with a transplanted kidney will develop proteinuria during the third trimester, which is not significant in the absence of hypertension (8). If any suspicion of preeclampsia exists, the patient should receive seizure prophylaxis. Patients treated with magnesium sulfate for preeclampsia should be closely monitored for magnesium toxicity as this drug is excreted via the kidneys. Fluid intake and urine output also should be monitored accurately. Continuous fetal monitoring should begin when the patient is admitted.

Immunosuppressive agents should be continued throughout labor and the postpartum period; both cyclosporine and azathioprine are available as injectable solutions. Consultation with transplant specialists is often helpful in adjusting a patient's drug regimen. Stress steroids are required if the patient has been on long-term therapy; 100 mg of hydrocortisone every 8 hours until 24 hours after delivery is most commonly used. Transplant patients are at an increased risk of infection due to the immunosuppression. Thus, the need for an intrauterine pressure catheter or urethral catheter should be carefully assessed because these increase the infectious risks. Davison and Lindheimer (9) recommended that any invasive procedure, including amniotomy or episiotomy, be accompanied by preprocedure prophylactic antibiotics. Chorioamnionitis and other infectious complications must be treated aggressively, but nephrotoxic antibiotics should be avoided.

Vaginal delivery is not contraindicated, and the transplanted kidney rarely obstructs labor. If there is suspicion of obstruction, limited intravenous pyelography with pelvimetry and ultrasonography can aid in making this diagnosis. Cesarean section should be reserved for standard obstetric indications, and the risk of adhesive disease from previous surgery or peritonitis should be kept in mind. Intravenous analgesia and regional anesthesia may be offered to patients without hesitation. In the event of cesarean delivery, nephrotoxic anesthetic agents should be avoided when possible.

■ REFERENCES

1. Anderson RJ, Linas SL, Berns AS, et al. Nonoliguric acute renal failure. N Engl J Med 1977;296:1134–1138.
2. Miller TR, Anderson RJ, Linas SL, et al. Urinary diagnostic indices in acute renal failure: a prospective study. Ann Intern Med 1978:89:47–50.
3. Lee W, Gonik B, Cotton DB. Urinary diagnostic indices in preeclampsia-associated oliguria: correlation with invasive hemodynamic monitoring. Am J Obstet Gynecol 1987;156:100–103.
4. Parker S, Carlon GC, Isaacs M, Howland WS, Kahn RC. Dopamine administration in oliguria and oliguric renal failure. Crit Care Med 1981;9:630–632.
5. Davison JM. Dialysis, transplantation and pregnancy. Am J Kidney Dis 1991;27:127.
6. Rizzoni G, Ehrich JHH, Broyen M, et al. Successful pregnancies in women on renal replacement therapy: report from EDTA registry. Nephrol Dial Transplant 1992;7:1.
7. Rudolph JE, Schweizer RT, Bar SA. Pregnancy in renal transplant patients. Transplantation 1979;27:26.
8. Penn I, Makowski EL, Harris P. Parenthood following renal transplantation. Kidney Int 1980;18:221.
9. Davison JM, Lindheimer MD. Renal disorders. In: Creasy RK, Resnik R, eds. Maternal-fetal medicine: principles and practice. 3rd ed. Philadelphia: WB Saunders Company, 1994:858.

Endocrine Disorders

▼ ▼ ▼ ▼ ▼

■ THYROID DISEASE

Hyperthyroidism

Hyperthyroidism complicates 0.2% of pregnancies and is most commonly caused by Graves' disease. Mild thyrotoxicosis is often difficult to detect as many of the symptoms overlap with those of normal pregnancy. However, a heart rate above 100 beats per minute, thyromegaly, exophthalmos, and failure of a nonobese woman to gain weight should raise suspicion of the disease. Although measuring the thyroid-stimulating hormone (TSH) level is a sensitive method to screen for the disease in nonpregnant patients, its usefulness as the sole screening test during pregnancy has not been confirmed. Therefore, a full thyroid panel (Table 6.1) should be considered in patients with symptoms of hyperthyroidism. Antepartum care involves treatment with propylthiouracil (PTU) or methimazole titrated to maintain thyroid function values in the normal range for pregnancy (Table 6.1). It is the untreated gravida who has an increased risk of intrapartum thyroid storm, congestive heart failure, preterm labor, preeclampsia, intrauterine growth restriction, and perinatal mortality. Neonatal thyrotoxicosis occurs in approximately 1% of infants born to

Table 6.1 *Effects of pregnancy and hyperthyroidism on thyroid function*

Parameter	Normal pregnancy[a]	Hyperthyroidism
TSH	No change	Decreased[b]
TBG	Increased	No change
Total T_4	Increased	Increased
Free T_4	No change	Increased
Total T_3	Increased	Increased
Free T_3	No change	Increased
T_3RU	Decreased	Increased

TSH = thyroid-stimulating hormone; TBG = thyroid-binding globulin; T_3RU = T_3 resin uptake.
[a]Compared to nonpregnant subjects.
[b]In rare cases of hyperthyroidism, TSH may be increased.

women with Graves' disease and may be manifested by a fetal heart rate faster than 160 beats per minute. This occurs independent of maternal treatment and is due to thyroid-stimulating antibody crossing the placenta. Since fetal goiter has been reported in infants whose mothers received an excessive amount of antithyroid medication during pregnancy, malpresentation of the fetus during labor should raise the suspicion of a fetal neck mass. Fetal bradycardia in the range of 110 beats per minute may also be suggestive of hypothyroidism.

When a patient presents in labor, it is important to be aware of the results of the most recent antenatal thyroid function tests, which will indicate the level of control. Confirmation that the patient has continued to take antepartum medications should be obtained. A patient whose disease is well controlled can be maintained on the antepartum drug regimen throughout labor and the postpartum period. Neither PTU nor methimazole are available in an injectable form, and therefore these medications can be taken during labor with sips of water at their usual dose and interval. Conversely, a patient who has not received antenatal medical therapy should be managed more aggressively since the risk of thyroid storm is increased. The drug regimen for these patients is similar to that for the patient in thyrotoxic crisis, as will be outlined.

Thyrotoxic Crisis

Thyrotoxic crisis (thyroid storm) has been reported to occur in 2% of patients who have received antithyroid medication and in 20% of those who have not received treatment during pregnancy (1). It is an acute exacerbation of inadequately treated thyrotoxicosis whereby the body's adaptive responses to the physiologic changes of hyperthyroidism can no longer compensate. In the majority of patients, a precipitating stress is present, including a serious infection (pneumonia, chorioamnionitis, sepsis, pyelonephritis), surgery, a thromboembolic event, preeclampsia, labor, molar pregnancy, an insulin reaction, or trauma. Patients with thyroid storm will present with signs and symptoms of hypermetabolism, as listed in Table 6.2. A normal body temperature in a patient with only mild anxiety should bring the diagnosis of thyroid storm into question. Arrhythmias and signs of congestive heart failure with pulmonary edema are more common in the untreated patient with thyro-

Table 6.2 *Signs and symptoms of thyroid storm*

Fever
Tachycardia > 140 beats/min
Diarrhea
Cutaneous vasodilation with heat intolerance
Warm moist extremities
Nervous anxiety to frank delirium and psychosis
Goiter
Exophthalmos
Arrhythmias
Congestive heart failure with pulmonary edema

toxicosis than in women with controlled disease. Patients may have a mild anemia, elevated white blood cell count, hyperglycemia, and abnormal liver enzyme levels, but none of these are required for the diagnosis. Furthermore, thyroid hormone levels do not distinguish patients with thyrotoxicosis from those with thyroid storm.

The successful management of thyroid storm is dependent on early and aggressive treatment, even if action is based on a presumptive diagnosis and laboratory evaluation is yet to be completed. Although a patient without thyroid storm may be overtreated, the risk-benefit ratio favors empiric treatment. The reported maternal mortality rate for thyroid storm once ranged from 30 to 100%, but more recently has been reduced to 10 to 20% (2).

An exhaustive search for precipitating factors must

be conducted early in the clinical course. Since the only laboratory evidence of infection may be an increased number of neutrophils despite a normal white blood cell count, a thorough examination for infection should be undertaken. Cultures of urine and blood should be obtained, and analysis of amniotic fluid may be clinically indicated. Other studies such as chest radiograph or spinal fluid analysis may be performed depending on the clinical picture.

The general management principles begin with intensive care surveillance of cardiac, pulmonary, and metabolic status. Body temperature control measures include a cooling blanket and rectal acetaminophen (600 mg every 3–4 hours). Aspirin should be avoided as it may inhibit thyroid hormone binding and thus increase circulating free hormone (3). When the patient's body temperature cannot be controlled with these measures, pharmacologic blockade can be achieved with 25 to 50 mg of intramuscular chlorpromazine. Intravenous fluids should be administered carefully, but often up to 4 liters of fluid is required in the initial 24 hours to compensate for losses due to fever and the increased metabolic state. Caloric requirements can be met partially by using intravenous solutions containing glucose. Respiratory insufficiency is relatively common in thyroid storm, and may be the result of pneumonia, congestive heart failure, or pulmonary embolism. Oxygen therapy should be titrated to maintain oxygen saturation above 95% by pulse oximetry.

In addition to these steps for stabilization of the maternal condition, specific goals in the medical management of thyroid storm include: 1) reversal of peripheral effects; 2) control of the synthesis and release of thyroid hormone; and 3) prevention or treatment of extreme hyperthermia, tachycardia, and cardiac arrhythmias (Table 6.3). The reversal of the peripheral actions of the thyroid hormones is achieved with beta-adrenergic antagonists. Propranolol has the advantage of being the only agent of this class with an inhibitory effect on the peripheral conversion of thyroxine (T_4) to triiodothyronine (T_3), thus reducing the amount of active thyroid hormone present in the peripheral circulation. The initial intravenous dose for severe tachycardia is 1 mg, which can be repeated every 5 minutes until the pulse rate is significantly decreased. An infusion at 5 to 10 mg/hour may then be initiated to maintain control of the heart rate. In less urgent situations, 40 to 80 mg of oral propranolol every 4 hours may be given. When the patient is afebrile, the heart rate should be maintained at 90 to 110 beats per minute. Control of tachycardia is often difficult in the febrile patient, and the heart rate may not respond to blocking doses of propranolol until the patient's body temperature has normalized. Beta blockers should not be administered to any patient with signs or symptoms of cardiac failure as these agents are myocardial depressants and may worsen the condition.

The drug regimen for reducing the synthesis and release of thyroid hormone includes the thioamides, iodides, and glucocorticoids. PTU or methimazole are the two thioamides employed to block the synthesis of thyroid hormone. However, these agents act slowly because they do not block the release of preformed hormone from the thyroid. PTU, but not methimazole, has the additional effect of blocking the peripheral conver-

Table 6.3 *Management of thyroid storm*

	Medication/treatment	Dose	Effect
Reversal of peripheral effects	Propylthiouracil (PTU)	600-mg oral load, then 300 mg every 6 hr	Inhibits conversion of T_4 to T_3
	Glucocorticoids (hydrocortisone)	100 mg IV every 8 hr	Inhibits conversion of T_4 to T_3
	Adrenergic antagonists (propranolol)	1 mg/min IV up to 10 mg every 4 hr *or* 40–80 mg orally every 4 hr	Inhibits conversion of T_4 to T_3
Control of the synthesis and release of thyroid hormone	PTU	(See above)	Inhibits iodination of tyrosine
	Methimazole	25 mg every 4 hr	Same as PTU
	Iodine therapy: Lugol's solution, sodium iodide, ipodate, or lithium carbonate		Inhibits proteolysis of thyroglobulin
	Glucocorticoids	(See above)	Uncertain
	Plasma exchange		Uncertain
Supportive measures	Acetaminophen		
	Cooling blankets		
	Chlorpromazine		
	Fluid replacement		
	Caloric replacement		
	Oxygen supplementation		
	Digoxin and diuretics for congestive heart failure		
	Glucocorticoids		

sion of T_4 to T_3, and is thus the preferred agent by many clinicians. The initial dose of PTU is 600 mg orally followed by 300 mg every 6 hours. Therapy with methimazole consists of 25 mg orally every 4 hours. Neither of these agents is available in injectable form and must be administered via a nasogastric tube if the patient is unable to take medications by mouth. The major side effect of both of these antithyroid medications is leukopenia.

Lugol's solution and saturated solution of potassium iodide (SSKI) act to quickly block hormone release from the thyroid and are available in most hospitals. The reported dosing regimen for Lugol's solution varies considerably, but one dose recommended is 8 drops (orally or by nasogastric tube) every 6 hours (4). SSKI can be administered in a manner similar to Lugol's solution. The problems of oral administration and the variable absorption rate can be avoided by using intravenous sodium iodide, 0.25 to 0.50 gm intravenously every 6 hours. This agent, however, may be difficult to obtain as it is used infrequently. Alternatively, an iodinated radiographic contrast dye such as ipodate sodium (e.g., Oragrafin) may be used when none of these three iodides are available. If a patient is allergic to iodine, 300 mg of lithium carbonate every 6 hours to achieve a therapeutic serum level (1 mEq/L) may be substituted. Long-term therapy with the iodides should be avoided owing to potential adverse fetal effects.

Glucocorticoids are important in the treatment of thyroid storm as they decrease the release of hormone from the thyroid and reduce the peripheral conversion of T_4 to T_3. These agents therefore have both a complementary and an additive effect with the actions of PTU.

Intravenous hydrocortisone is administered at a dose of 100 mg every 8 hours. Dexamethasone (2 mg given intramuscularly or by mouth, depending on the severity of illness) is an alternative therapy, but it holds no particular advantage.

Congestive heart failure is a life-threatening complication of untreated hyperthyroidism and thyrotoxic crisis. Diuresis is initiated with intravenous furosemide at a dose of 20 to 40 mg. The heart rate in patients with congestive failure can be controlled with intravenous digoxin, 0.5 mg given over 5 minutes followed by two doses of 0.25 mg at 4- to 8-hour intervals. Due to the patient's increased metabolic rate, higher doses of this agent may be required to achieve the therapeutic levels of 1 to 2 ng/mL as measured by most laboratories.

Understanding the underlying pathophysiology of thyroid storm is critical in avoiding therapeutic pitfalls (5). Maintenance of intravascular volume to prevent vasoconstriction and allow peripheral heat dissipation is important despite the potential need for diuretics. The patient's body temperature should be lowered at a rate so as to avoid shivering, which is induced by rapid cooling. In addition to congestive heart failure, beta blockers should not be administered to patients with moderate to severe asthma because this can result in bronchoconstriction. Patients whose tachycardia is secondary to infection-related fever may not respond as well to beta blockers as patients without underlying infection. Beta-adrenergic agents should not be administered for tocolysis as this will only potentiate the complications of thyroid storm.

Optimally, delivery for the patient with thyroid

storm should await maternal stabilization. Although continuous fetal monitoring should be instituted on admission, surgical intervention must await clear evidence of fetal distress. Fetal tachycardia can result from maternal pyrexia and the hypermetabolic state. Severe dehydration leading to relative uteroplacental insufficiency can be corrected with appropriate fluid management. Early consultation with an anesthesiologist and neonatologist is essential for comprehensive patient care. There is no contraindication to vaginal delivery, and the maternal morbidity associated with cesarean delivery is significantly increased.

Hypothyroidism

Hypothyroidism may result from a variety of etiologies, including surgically treated or radioiodine-treated Graves' disease and Hashimoto's thyroiditis. The typical presentation of a patient with hypothyroidism is described in Table 6.4. Laboratory evaluation reveals an abnormally elevated TSH and a decreased free T_4 level.

Table 6.4 *Signs and symptoms of hypothyroidism*

Fatigue

Cold intolerance

Hair loss

Dry skin

Constipation

Delayed deep tendon reflexes

Patients whose thyroid function is normalized as a result of levothyroxine frequently achieve pregnancy, which is in contrast to the infertility often associated with untreated hypothyroidism. There is little information regarding the outcome of pregnancy in women with subclinical hypothyroidism (elevated TSH with normal T_4 and T_3 levels) and treated hypothyroidism. In general, the infants of women with treated disease appear to be healthy. However, Davis et al (6) reported on the increased incidence of preeclampsia, abruptio placentae, postpartum hemorrhage, low-birth-weight infants, and stillbirths in women with overt, untreated hypothyroidism.

When a patient with a history of hypothyroidism presents in labor, the most recent antenatal thyroid function test results should be available to determine whether the patient is euthyroid. The intrapartum management of the patient with adequately treated hypothyroidism does not differ from standard care. Since levothyroxine has a serum half-life of 1 week, withholding one to two scheduled doses during labor will not affect the patient's clinical status.

Untreated hypothyroidism may result in myxedema with a clinical picture of an expressionless face, sparse hair, large tongue, pale and cool skin, and periorbital swelling. Adynamic ileus with or without megacolon, prolonged relaxation phase of deep tendon reflexes, cardiac enlargement, or pericardial effusion may be present in these patients. Myxedema coma may ultimately develop, and is characterized by hypothermia, decreased mentation, respiratory depression, and eventually cardiovascular collapse.

General supportive measures in a patient with severe, untreated hypothyroidism or myxedema include maintenance of body temperature, intravenous fluid management, and antibiotic therapy if infection is suspected. Most patients will require only blankets to reduce heat loss and maintain body temperature. Excessive warming will result in peripheral vasodilation and can lead to cardiovascular shock. It has been suggested that external warming measures be instituted when the body temperature is less than 30°C (5). Intravenous fluids should contain glucose as needed to maintain euglycemia. Hypothyroid patients are also very susceptible to water intoxication, and administration of saline solution may be required to maintain a serum sodium level in the normal range (7). Antibiotic therapy should be initiated early in the course of suspected infection, and is guided by the presumed source.

Impaired respiratory function may result from a reduced central drive to hypoxia and hypercarbia, weakened respiratory muscles, or concurrent pulmonary infection. There is also evidence that surfactant production in the lung is decreased in myxedema (8). Therefore, even with ventilatory support, hypercarbia but not hypoxia may be corrected. In addition, the patient with myxedema often has anemia that may worsen the hypoxia and oxygen delivery. Pulse oximetry may be employed to monitor a patient's pulmonary status, but arterial blood gas analysis should be performed for more accurate assessment if there is any evidence of pulmonary compromise or a saturation less than 95%. Endotracheal intubation and mechanical ventilation must not be delayed if the patient shows signs of pulmonary insufficiency, as rapid deterioration and irreversible shock may ensue without respiratory assistance.

The cardiovascular adaptations to the decreased thermogenesis of hypothyroidism include marked peripheral vasoconstriction secondary to relatively unopposed alpha-adrenergic stimulation. The intravascular volume of a patient with myxedema is generally reduced by approximately 1 liter and this may be due to peripheral vasoconstriction. Excessive warming measures with resultant vasodilation, gastrointestinal bleeding with hypotension, or sepsis may further contribute to the decreased intravascular volume.

Medical therapy for the correction of myxedema coma includes levothyroxine and steroids. Thyroid function tests should be performed prior to starting levothyroxine, but hormonal therapy should not be withheld while awaiting these results. Levothyroxine is available as an injectable form and is administered at a dose of 300 $\mu g/m^2$. Glucocorticoid administration has been empirically recommended to compensate for a relative adrenal insufficiency as a normal metabolic state is restored (5,9). Since scant data are available regarding the acute management of this uncommon condition in pregnancy, few specific recommendations can be made pertaining to intrapartum care.

■ DIABETES

Gestational Diabetes

Gestational diabetes affects 60,000 to 100,000 pregnancies per year in the United States. The strict definition includes patients diagnosed with diabetes for the first time during pregnancy (10). In practice, however, a patient with pregestational diabetes may be initially diagnosed antenatally. Because untreated diabetes is associated with increased perinatal morbidity and mortality, universal screening of all pregnant women for gestational diabetes is advocated. Even with adequate control of maternal glucose levels, the patient remains at risk for macrosomia and polyhydramnios and neonates may suffer from hypoglycemia, hypocalcemia, polycythemia, and hyperbilirubinemia. The maternal effects of gestational diabetes are primarily related to trauma associated with a difficult delivery, an increased rate of cesarean section due to macrosomia, and a higher risk of recurrent gestational diabetes as well as overt diabetes in later life (11–13).

The gravida with gestational diabetes may be allowed to go into spontaneous labor at term providing glucose control is adequate and there are no other complicating factors such as preeclampsia, intrauterine growth restriction, chronic hypertension, or macrosomia. Ultrasonographic estimation of fetal weight should ideally be performed near term to assist in determining the mode of delivery. Although ultrasonography has a 10 to 20% margin of error in estimating fetal weight, the American College of Obstetricians and Gynecologists recommends elective cesarean delivery when the fetus of a gestational diabetic has an estimated weight higher than 4500 gm (14). The decision to perform a cesarean section for macrosomia or any specific birth-weight category remains controversial and must be individualized.

A woman with gestational diabetes whose glycemic control has been maintained by diet alone during pregnancy should have serial capillary blood glucose determinations during labor. A glucose reflectance meter is ideal for this purpose and is generally available in the hospital setting. The type of intravenous fluid infused during labor is of minor importance, and may be determined based on maternal glucose levels. Although most patients whose diabetes has been controlled by diet do not require intrapartum insulin, the protocol outlined for the insulin-dependent diabetic should be instituted if the blood glucose concentration is higher than 120 mg/dL. A gestational diabetic who has required insulin for glycemic control antenatally is also managed during labor the way the patient with insulin-dependent diabetes is.

As previously mentioned, the patient with gestational diabetes is at increased risk for shoulder dystocia. A complete discussion of this obstetric complication is beyond the scope of this text, and can be found in a variety of standard obstetric references. Briefly, shoulder dystocia remains a condition that is difficult to predict prior to its occurrence. Although various risk factors, including abnormalities in labor progression and midpelvic operative procedures, have been suggested, their utility in the clinical setting remains uncertain. The obstetrician caring for a diabetic patient must have a high index of suspicion for the potential occurrence of shoulder dystocia, and should be skilled in the various maneuvers required to alleviate this condition.

Postpartum, a patient with gestational diabetes who has not required insulin may resume a regular dietary intake. Fasting and 2-hour postprandial blood glucose levels should be measured on the first postpartum day. If the patient has delivered by cesarean section and remains on intravenous fluids, serial capillary glucose determinations can be obtained to ensure a euglycemic state. At discharge, the patient should be counseled regarding the need for a 75-gm glucose tolerance test as recommended by the National Diabetes Data Group (15).

Insulin-Dependent Diabetes

The outcome of pregnancies complicated by insulin-dependent diabetes mellitus has significantly improved since the discovery of insulin in 1922. However, the perinatal mortality rate among women with diabetes remains twice that of their nondiabetic counterparts (15). Congenital malformations, intrauterine fetal demise, and respiratory distress syndrome are responsible for most of the perinatal deaths associated with diabetes. Macrosomia and intrapartum asphyxia remain significant causes of neonatal morbidity and mortality. The neonates of women with insulin-dependent diabetes are also at risk of suffering from the same metabolic and hematologic complications as the infant of gravidas with gestational diabetes.

Depending on the duration of the disease, women with preexisting insulin-dependent diabetes are at risk for various medical and obstetric complications. The effect of diabetes on the ophthalmologic, renal, and cardiovascular systems must be assessed antenatally and abnormalities followed for progression. Chronic hypertension, preeclampsia, abruptio placentae, and stroke occur more frequently in patients with evidence of retinal or renal vasculopathy (16–19). Women with type I diabetes remain at risk for diabetic ketoacidosis, which can occur at a blood glucose level significantly less than that in the nonpregnant patient (20).

Table 6.5 *Insulin therapy during labor*

Obtain capillary blood glucose level at admission

Start 5–10% dextrose intravenous solution at 125 ml/hr

Insulin infusion

    Prepare 25 units of regular insulin in 250 mL of normal saline (1 U/10 mL)

    Begin 0.5 U/hr (5 mL/hr) of insulin infusion if glucose level > 120 mg/dL

Determine capillary blood glucose level hourly or with symptoms of hypoglycemia

Increase insulin infusion by 0.5–1.0 U/hr to maintain glucose level of 60–120 mg/dL

Dip urine for ketones every 4–6 hr (if present with euglycemia, suspect starvation ketosis)

Patients with well-controlled blood glucose levels can be allowed to go into spontaneous labor at term, providing antenatal fetal surveillance has been reassuring. When induction of labor is indicated for medical or obstetric reasons and the cervix is unfavorable, prostaglandin gel may be used for ripening as it has no adverse effects on glycemic control. The patient may continue her routine diabetic diet and antenatal insulin regimen with blood glucose testing while she is receiving the gel. An elevated glucose level may be treated with intermittent injections of subcutaneous regular insulin. When a contraction pattern is established, the protocol for intravenous glucose and insulin should be initiated (Table 6.5).

Patients with a favorable cervix in whom induction

of labor will be started with oxytocin should refrain from eating after midnight and be instructed to take one half of their morning insulin dose on the day of induction. After blood glucose concentration is measured, an intravenous glucose solution should be started immediately on admission to the labor and delivery unit. Insulin therapy can then be instituted as outlined in Table 6.5.

Maintenance of maternal glucose control and avoidance of ketoacidosis are important in order to avoid intrapartum fetal compromise and acidosis. However, the neonate may still suffer from metabolic aberrations in the nursery despite adequate maternal glycemic control during labor. Two methods of insulin administration that have been described include a continuous intravenous infusion and intermittent subcutaneous injections (21). The primary benefit of a continuous infusion is the ease with which maternal glucose levels can be regulated. Regardless of the treatment regimen chosen, maternal glucose determinations must be made on an hourly basis throughout labor. It is important to remember that insulin requirements have been shown to decrease significantly during the active phase of labor (22), and thus the insulin infusion rate may need to be lowered as labor progresses.

Postpartum, the patient with type I diabetes whose blood glucose concentration has been difficult to control during labor may be continued on an insulin drip until a glucose range of 150 to 200 mg/dL is achieved. Otherwise, women who have had a vaginal delivery may resume their pregestational diabetic diet and sliding-scale coverage until the next morning. On the morning of the first postpartum day, one third to one half of the prepregnancy insulin dose may be administered, with sliding-scale coverage for the remainder of the day. The total units of insulin required during the first day may be used as a guide to divide the insulin dose for subsequent days. If a patient with type I diabetes has undergone a cesarean section, the insulin infusion may be continued or intermittent subcutaneous insulin initiated. As the patient's diet is advanced, the total number of units required in the preceding 24 hours may be used as a guide in prescribing the insulin regimen for the next 12 to 24 hours. In the patient with poorly controlled diabetes who has had an operative delivery, it is important to optimize wound care since hyperglycemia and vascular disease impair healing.

Patients with insulin-requiring gestational diabetes generally do not require insulin following delivery. Capillary blood glucose determinations should be performed prior to and 2 hours after meals to assess the need for insulin. A woman who continues to have elevated blood glucose levels after delivery may indeed have pregestational diabetes that was undiagnosed before pregnancy and will benefit from follow-up care with a primary care physician.

■ REFERENCES

1. Davis LE, Lucas MJ, Hankins GDV, Roark ML, Cunningham FG. Thyrotoxicosis complicating pregnancy. Am J Obstet Gynecol 1989;160:63–70.
2. Singer PA, Mestman JH. Thyroid storm need not be lethal. Contemp Obstet Gynecol 1983;135–146.
3. Larsen PR. Salicylate-induced increases in free triiodothyronine in human serum. J Clin Invest 1972;51:1125.

4. Branch DW. Thyroid storm. Contemp Obstet Gynecol 1994;4:11–20.

5. Nicoloff JT. Thyroid storm and myxedema coma. Med Clin North Am 1985;69:1005–1017.

6. Davis LE, Leveno KJ, Cunningham FG. Hypothyroidism complicating pregnancy. Obstet Gynecol 1988;72:108–12.

7. Pettinger WA, Talner L, Ferris TF. Inappropriate secretion of antidiuretic hormone due to myxedema. N Engl J Med 1965;272:362–364.

8. Redding RA, Douglas WH. Thyroid hormone influence upon lung surfactant metabolism. Science 1972;175:994–996.

9. Reed Larson P. The thyroid. In: Wyngaarden JB, Smith LH, eds. Cecil textbook of medicine. Philadelphia: WB Saunders Company, 1988:1328–1331.

10. Dickinson JE, Palmer SM. Gestational diabetes. Semin Perinatol 1990;14:2–11.

11. O'Sullivan JB. Body weight and subsequent diabetes mellitus. JAMA 1982;248:949.

12. Oats JN, Beischer NA. The persistence of abnormal glucose tolerance after delivery. Obstet Gynecol 1990;75:397.

13. Philipson EH, Super DM. Gestational diabetes mellitus: does it recur in subsequent pregnancy? Am J Obstet Gynecol 1989;160:1324.

14. Fetal macrosomia. ACOG Technical Bulletin No. 159. American College of Obstetricians and Gynecologists, Washington, DC, September 1991.

15. Landon MB. Diabetes mellitus and other endocrine diseases. In: Gabbe SG, Niebyl JR, Simpson JL, eds. 2nd ed. Obstetrics: normal and problem pregnancies. New York: Churchill Livingstone, 1991:1097.

16. Combs CA, Rosenn B, Kitzmiller JL, et al. Early-pregnancy proteinuria in diabetes related to preeclampsia. Obstet Gynecol 1993;82:802–807.

17. Reece EA, Coustan DR, Hayslett JP, et al. Diabetic nephropathy: pregnancy performance and fetomaternal outcome. Am J Obstet Gynecol 1988;159:56.

18. Knowler WC, Bennett PH, Ballintine EJ. Increased incidence of diabetic retinopathy in diabetics with elevated blood pressure: a six year follow-up in Pima Indians. N Engl J Med 1980;302:645–650.

19. Kornerup T. Studies in diabetic retinopathy: an investigation of 1000 cases of diabetics. Acta Med Scand 1955; 153:83–101.

20. Montoro MN, Myers VP, Mestman JH, Yunhua X, Anderson BG, Golde SH. Outcome of pregnancy in diabetic ketoacidosis. Am J Perinatol 1993;10:17–20.

21. Yudkin JS, Knopfler A. Glucose and insulin infusions during labour. Lancet 1992;339:1479.

22. Jovanovic L, Peterson CM. Management of the pregnant, insulin-dependent diabetic woman. Diabetes Care 1980;3: 63.

Hematologic Disease

▼   ▼   ▼   ▼   ▼

■ IRON DEFICIENCY ANEMIA

Iron deficiency anemia is the most common cause of anemia during pregnancy. Since the fetus preferentially absorbs iron, women with marginal iron stores will very quickly become iron deficient during pregnancy. Patients may complain of excessive fatigue, lethargy, and headache. Laboratory findings include a microcytic, hypochromic anemia with low plasma iron and serum ferritin levels. Ideally, patients will have received iron supplementation throughout pregnancy, but some gravidas enter labor with a significant anemia as a result of iron deficiency.

Patients with long-standing anemia have generally adjusted to a given hemoglobin level and tolerate their anemia better than the patient who suffers from an acute loss as with hemorrhage. Hemoglobin/hematocrit should be determined and type and crossmatch obtained at admission to labor and delivery. The number of units of packed red blood cells ordered will depend on the patient's blood cell count and the clinical situation, but a minimum of 2 units should be available since most obstetric hemorrhage is not predictable. Adequate oxygenation should be ensured throughout labor, and continuous fetal monitoring instituted on the patient's arrival. Although notoriously difficult to estimate, careful attention must be given to any intrapartum blood loss (1,2).

If excessive blood loss was noted at delivery, hemoglobin/hematocrit should be determined in the recovery room. However, it must be kept in mind that several hours may be required for equilibration to occur. Transfusion of packed red blood cells is indicated for any hemodynamically unstable patient, and should be strongly considered if the hemoglobin is less than 6 gm/dL or hematocrit is less than 18%. Hemoglobin/hematocrit determined on the first postpartum day will most accurately reflect the patient's hemoglobin level. Iron supplementation for 2 to 6 months postpartum should be recommended to replenish the patient's depleted iron stores.

■ SICKLE CELL TRAIT

Patients with sickle cell trait (SCT) generally tolerate pregnancy with minimal difficulty. The diagnosis is based on a positive screening test with confirmation by hemoglobin electrophoresis (Table 7.1). An important concern in the preconceptional or antenatal care of the woman with SCT is the genetic aspect of being a carrier of the sickle trait. Since gravidas with SCT are at an increased risk for lower urinary tract infection and pyelonephritis (3,4), routine surveillance during pregnancy is recommended. The main consideration during labor is maintenance of adequate oxygenation as significant hypoxia may result in sickling of red blood cells. There is no contraindication to epidural anesthesia or vaginal delivery in the woman with sickle trait.

Table 7.1 *Hemoglobin electrophoresis in the diagnosis of hemoglobinopathies*

	Electrophoresis characteristics				
Common diagnoses	HbA	HbS	HbA$_2$	HbF	HbC
Sickle cell trait	55–60%	40–45%	2–3%	1%	0%
Sickle cell disease*	0%	85–95%	2–3%	5–15%	0%
Hemoglobin SC*	0%	45–50%	2–3%	1%	45–50%
Beta thalassemia trait	90–95%	0%	4–8%	1–3%	0%

*In patients not recently transfused.

■ SICKLE CELL DISEASE

Sickle cell disease (SCD), an autosomal recessive condition with a characteristic hemoglobin electrophoresis, may affect any organ system of the body (see Table 7.1). A significant reduction in solubility in deoxygenated states and a markedly shortened life span of red blood cells are hallmarks of this chronic disease. The majority of the clinical manifestations of SCD are the result of hemolysis, vaso-occlusive disease, or an increased susceptibility to infection (Table 7.2). A vaso-occlusive pain crisis may be precipitated by hypoxia, infection, pregnancy, cold, or alcohol consumption. The course of SCD during pregnancy varies between individuals, with the most common antepartum concerns including pain crisis, pulmonary complications from infection and embolization, and congestive heart failure. Painful crisis may be more common during the intrapartum period secondary to the increased oxygen demands (5).

Hemoglobin/hematocrit should be determined and a type and crossmatch obtained at admission. The number of packed red blood cells made available may be determined based on the initial blood study results and other clinical factors. The issue of prophylactic and partial exchange transfusions remains controversial, and practices vary by institution (6–10).

The intrapartum management of a patient with SCD emphasizes adequate oxygenation, hydration and pain control, continuous fetal monitoring, and avoidance of a pain crisis. The patient should be placed on her left side in a warm, quiet, comfortable environment. Supplemental oxygen should be administered to minimize the

Table 7.2 *Common clinical findings of sickle cell anemia*

Sickle cell crisis

Abdominal, bone, chest, and back pain

Cardiac

Systolic murmur

Congestive heart failure

Cardiomegaly

Pulmonary

Chest syndrome

Pneumonia

Infarction

Abdominal

Painful vascular occlusion

Cholelithiasis/cholecystitis

Hepatomegaly

Splenic infarction

Hepatitis

Genitourinary

Pyelonephritis

Hematuria

Neurologic

Cerebral ischemia

Cerebral hemorrhage

Visual changes

Seizures

chance of hypoxia, which may precipitate a pain crisis. A crystalloid intravenous solution may be infused at a maintenance rate, with urine output being monitored as an indicator of the patient's renal perfusion. Narcotics should be used liberally to control labor pain. In the patient with a history of frequent crises, larger than expected doses of narcotics may be required owing to drug tolerance. There is no contraindication to regional anesthesia for labor and delivery (11), but hypotension and resultant uterine hypoperfusion should be avoided.

Continuous fetal monitoring allows optimal surveillance of a fetus subject to chronic hypoxia or growth restriction. It should be remembered that fetal heart rate tracings may be more difficult to interpret in the patient who requires a higher than the usual dosage of a narcotic agent. Since use of a fetal scalp electrode and intrauterine pressure catheter may increase the risk of infection, they should be placed only when clearly indicated. Although universal intrapartum prophylactic antibiotics are not beneficial to SCD patients, aggressive therapy with these agents, following appropriate culturing, is recommended when infection is suspected. As with any other obstetric patient, prophylactic antibiotics may be required for cesarean delivery or prevention of subacute bacterial endocarditis.

In the event a pain crisis develops during labor, a careful search for the precipitating factor must be made. The principles for treatment of a crisis include adequate oxygenation, pain relief, and hydration. Transfusion of packed red blood cells may be required for the patient with a hemoglobin level less than 8 gm/dL. Since these patients maintain a relatively normal intravascular volume, a slow transfusion rate or the use of furosemide should be considered to minimize the risk of fluid overload. Delivery should be effected in a timely fashion with assurance of adequate fetal oxygenation through continuous fetal heart rate monitoring.

The mode of delivery is unaffected by the presence of SCD, and vaginal delivery is preferred. There is no contraindication to general anesthesia for cesarean section in patients with SCD if a regional block provides inadequate anesthesia or emergent delivery is required. During the initial postpartum period, the patient remains at risk for thromboembolism and vaso-occlusive crisis. Therefore, early ambulation and at times, heparin prophylaxis are indicated. The frequency of pulmonary complications reportedly is increased in patients who require endotracheal intubation for delivery, and careful attention to pulmonary toilet is required.

Contraceptive counseling is complicated by the fact that oral contraceptives are relatively contraindicated owing to the presumptive increased risk of thrombosis. Likewise, an intrauterine device is not recommended due to the risks associated with pelvic infection. Some clinicians advocate intramuscular medroxyprogesterone acetate suspension or levonorgestrel implants as methods of contraception for these women. Alternatively, barrier methods such as condoms, diaphragms, and spermicides are commonly recommended.

■ HEMOGLOBIN SC DISEASE

Hemoglobin SC disease (HbSC) is found in women who are doubly heterozygous for the hemoglobin S and C genes. The clinical manifestations of HbSC are similar to those of SCD but are less severe. However, patients with HbSC experience severe anemic crises due to splenic sequestration of the deformed erythrocytes. In addition, bone marrow necrosis and release of fat-forming emboli are seen in these patients (12). The management of patients with HbSC disease is similar to that of patients with SCD as previously outlined.

■ THALASSEMIAS

The thalassemias are a group of genetic diseases with a defect in the production of one or more of the polypeptide globin chains. There is a corresponding decrease in the amount of hemoglobin synthesized with an excess of normal globin chains. The classification of the thalassemias is based on the deficient globin production, alpha and beta being most common. A woman and her partner can be easily screened for thalassemia by examining the red blood cell indices obtained with a complete blood cell count. Remarkable indices include a decreased mean cell volume and mean corpuscular hemoglobin concentration, while the hemoglobin level may be normal or a mild hypochromic, microcytic anemia may be present. Hemoglobin electrophoresis may be used to confirm the carrier status and identify the deficient globin chain (see Table 7.1).

Beta Thalassemia

Beta thalassemia is the most common type of thalassemia and is found most often in individuals of Mediterranean descent. The homozygous form (beta thalassemia major) results in a severe, transfusion-dependent anemia, and patients generally do not survive beyond the third decade of life. It is rare that a woman with beta thalassemia major becomes pregnant; thus data are extremely limited.

Patients who are heterozygous for the disease, lacking only one beta-globin gene, are usually asymptomatic with normal findings on physical examination. Women who are carriers for this disease do not suffer any adverse effects during pregnancy, with the exception of a slightly lower hemoglobin. There are no specific considerations for the intrapartum and postpartum care of these patients.

Alpha Thalassemia

Alpha thalassemia is a rare disease found in people from Southeast China and the Mediterranean. The complete lack of alpha-globin chain synthesis is lethal, and thus prenatal diagnosis is of utmost importance for the gravida and her partner who are heterozygous for this condition. Women who have one or two of the four alpha-globin genes do not have any complications of pregnancy secondary to their carrier status.

■ TRANSFUSION THERAPY

Pregnant patients most frequently require transfusion of blood and blood products as a result of an obstetric complication during labor or following delivery. Since this text concentrates on the management of medical complications of pregnancy, the discussion in this section is limited to the general principles and complications of transfusion therapy. The management of specific obstetric events with hemorrhagic complications is not addressed individually.

Generally, the need for transfusion in obstetric patients cannot be anticipated. Any patient undergoing an operative procedure or admitted for labor should have at minimum a type and screen. A type and cross-match should be ordered for patients in whom the need for transfusion is increased. Women who have had a cesarean section, those with multiple gestation, placenta previa, or coagulation disorder, and those receiving an anticoagulant are at increased risk of requiring a transfusion, but this risk is neither absolute nor predictable. Although autologous transfusion has gained popularity, it is not considered practical or cost-effective for the majority of obstetric patients (13–16).

The goals of transfusion therapy are: 1) improvement of oxygen transport, 2) correction of coagulation abnormalities, and 3) restoration of circulatory volume. Correction of the underlying cause of the hemorrhage is paramount while the need for transfusion is being assessed. Clinical assessment of blood loss is frequently difficult, and signs of hypovolemic shock may not be present until 20% of blood volume has been lost. The degree of hemorrhage can be classified based on estimated volume loss and associated clinical signs (Table 7.3). Urinary output provides an accurate indication of renal perfusion and should always be carefully monitored in the patient with hypovolemia secondary to hemorrhage.

The initial treatment of hemorrhagic shock includes establishing intravenous access with large-bore catheters and administering crystalloid aggressively (3 mL of crystalloid per 1 mL of blood loss). Some investigators (17) recommend 5% albumin or 67% hetastarch for initial

Table 7.3 Classification of hemorrhage

	Blood loss (mL)	% Blood volume	Heart rate (beats per minute)	Blood pressure	Urine output
Class I	750–900	15–20	< 100	Normal	Normal
Class II	900–1500	20–30	< 100	Mild hypotension	Normal
Class III	1500–2000	30–40	100–120	Hypotension	Oliguria
Class IV	> 2000	> 40%	> 120	< 60 mm Hg	Anuria

replacement therapy. Indications for transfusion, contents of components, and the effects of packed red blood cells, platelets, fresh frozen plasma, and cryoprecipitate are summarized in Table 7.4 (18).

When the situation allows, patients who require administration of blood products should be counseled regarding the associated risks. Complications associated with transfusion therapy can be classified as infectious, immunologic, and mechanical. Massive transfusion is not strictly defined, but is often considered to be replacement of the patient's entire blood volume (5000 mL or approximately 10 units of packed red blood cells) in a 24-hour period (19). Complications specific to administration of significant quantities of red blood cells include hyperkalemia, citrate toxicity, volume overload, acidosis, and dilutional coagulopathy.

As donor and component screening has become more elaborate, the incidence of noninfectious transfusion-associated reactions has exceeded that for infectious complications. Although many patients perceive the acquired immunodeficiency syndrome (AIDS) as the most significant risk of receiving blood products, other transfusion-associated infections are more common (Table 7.5) (20). All donated blood is screened for hepatitis B and C viruses, syphilis, human immunodeficiency virus types 1 and 2 (HIV-1 and -2), and human T-cell lymphotropic virus types I and II (HTLV-I and -II).

The most serious of the immunologic complications is an acute hemolytic reaction due to transfusion of incompatible packed red blood cells. Rarely, this reaction is seen with administration of platelets, fresh frozen plasma, or cryoprecipitate. In the acute hemolytic reac-

Table 7.4 *Transfusion therapy*

Component	Contents	Volume	Indication for use	Results
Packed red blood cells	Red blood cells (RBCs) Contaminant white blood cells (WBCs) Platelet fragments	250 mL	Anemia	Increases hematocrit 3%/unit and hemoglobin 1gm/dL/U
Platelets	Minimum 5.5×10^{10} platelets/U Contaminant RBCs and WBCs	50–70 mL/U	Prophylactic for < 10–$20,000/mm^3$ platelets $< 50,000/mm^3$ platelets with active bleeding, *or* Operative procedure	Increases platelet count 5–10,000/mm^3/U

Fresh frozen plasma	Coagulation factors Fibrinogen, factors II, XIII Regulatory proteins Antithrombin III, plasminogen, protein C and S	200–250 ml/U	Correction of coagulopathy Reverse coumarin effect Correct factor deficiency when specific concentrate unavailable Treat TTP and HUS	Increases fibrinogen 10 dL/U
Cryoprecipitate	Factors VIII:C, XIII Von Willebrand factor 200–300 mg of fibrinogen	10–15 mL/U	Hemophilia A Von Willebrand's disease Hypofibrinogenemia Factor XIII deficiency Fibrin glue	Increases fibrinogen 10 dL/U

TTP = thrombotic thrombocytopenic purpura; HUS = hemolytic-uremic syndrome.

tion, the patient has antibodies to red blood cell antigens (most commonly ABO), resulting in rapid destruction of the transfused red blood cells. Formation of the antigen-antibody complex results in complement fixation, and the release of complement fragments. Cytokines released by the activation of the complement cascade contribute to the symptom complex. Acute hemolytic transfusion reactions can result in renal failure, shock, disseminated intravascular coagulation, and death.

Initial treatment of the reaction includes prompt recognition of the syndrome and stopping the transfusion (Table 7.6). Donor identification numbers should be verified as clerical error is the most common reason for this adverse reaction. A venous blood sample must be obtained from the patient and sent to the blood bank with the blood component product for repeat crossmatch. Close attention must be given to obtaining additional laboratory studies, maintaining adequate urine output, and observing for evidence of coagulopathy (see Table 7.6). Some clinicians would prophylactically

Table 7.5 *Transfusion-associated risks*

Complication	Risk/screened unit
Febrile reaction	1–3:100
Hepatitis C virus	1:3300
Acute hemolytic reaction	1:20,000
Human T-cell lymphotropic virus type I	1:50,000
Hepatitis B virus	1:200,000
Human immunodeficiency virus	1:250,000

Table 7.6 *Signs, symptoms, and management of acute hemolytic reaction*

Clinical features

  Fever

  Chills

  Back pain

  Dyspnea

  Tachycardia

  Hypotension

  Bronchospasm

  Hemoglobinuria

  Hemoglobinemia

  Disseminated intravascular coagulopathy

Initial treatment

  Stop blood product infusion

  Verification of donor identification numbers

  Venous blood sample and blood product for repeat
    crossmatch

  Obtain baseline fibrinogen, PT, PTT, and platelet count (repeat
    at 12 and 24 hr if initially normal)

  Serum sample for free hemoglobin (pink coloration) or
    methemalbuminemia (brown coloration)

  Intravenous hydration to maintain urine output of
    approximately 100 mL/hr

  Urine sample for free hemoglobin

  Consider pharmacologic diuresis

  Platelets, fresh frozen plasma, and cryoprecipitate as indicated
    to correct coagulopathy

PT = prothrombin time; PTT = partial thromboplastin time.

administer furosemide, 20 to 40 mg intravenously, to maintain urine output. In the event that more aggressive diuresis with an agent such as mannitol is required, or acute tubular necrosis develops, consultation with a renal specialist is needed.

Febrile nonhemolytic transfusion reactions are due to antibodies to leukocyte antigens found on the white blood cells contained within cellular blood components (packed red blood cells and platelets). Removal of the contaminating leukocytes reduces the incidence of febrile reactions. Allergic reactions may occur in response to plasma proteins in the unit of platelets, fresh frozen plasma, cryoprecipitate, or red blood cells. Patients can develop pruritis, bronchospasm, laryngospasm, anaphylaxis, and even death. Initial treatment is symptomatic relief with 25 to 50 mg of intravenous or oral diphenhydramine, but intravenous steroids are required for severe cases.

Mechanical complications of blood product transfusion include hypothermia and intravascular volume overload. Hypothermia is due to rapid infusion of packed red blood cell units (4°C) or freshly thawed fresh frozen plasma that have not been warmed. Transfusion of 6 or more units of cold packed cells has also been associated with ventricular arrhythmias and cardiac arrest (21). Additional advantages of warming the units include decreased viscosity and venous dilation. Since blood components are an excellent source of intravascular volume expansion, careful attention to the patient's fluid status is important. Intravenous furosemide (20 mg) administered prior to or during component infusion will minimize the risk of volume overload in patients at

risk for pulmonary edema. However, circulatory overload may occur at any time during the initial 24 hours
following the transfusion.

■ THE ANTICOAGULATED GRAVIDA

The indication for anticoagulation during pregnancy
varies but is most frequently a history of thromboembolism. The antiphospholipid antibody syndrome, presence of a mechanical heart valve, and an underlying
defect of the fibrinolytic or anticoagulant systems are
additional reasons why a gravida may require anticoagulation. The regimens vary among clinicians, and discussed here is just one approach to the intrapartum care
of the anticoagulated patient.

Heparin is the most commonly used anticoagulant
during pregnancy, because it does not cross the placenta.
The half-life of intravenous heparin is approximately 60
minutes, and the typical goal of therapy is to achieve an
activated partial thromboplastin time (aPTT) of 1.5 to 2.0
times the patient's baseline value. Heparin levels may be
measured instead of the aPTT, with a therapeutic range
of 0.2 to 0.4 unit/mL. The maternal risks of heparin use
include bleeding, heparin-induced thrombocytopenia
with paradoxical maternal thrombosis, and bone demin-
eralization with extended use.

Coumarin derivatives have a lower molecular
weight and easily cross the placenta. The half-life of coumarin is much longer than that of heparin, and its action
may persist for as long as 5 days. First-trimester use of
coumarin is associated with fetal embryopathy whereas
use later in pregnancy can result in fetal coagulopathy. Oral anticoagulants are administered to pregnant

patients with a contraindication to heparin (e.g., heparin-induced thrombocytopenia). Hemorrhagic complications are the greatest risk of coumarin therapy.

When *prophylactic* heparin (5000–8000 units given subcutaneously twice daily) is utilized during the antepartum period, withholding therapy once active labor begins is reasonable. Alternatively, the heparin may be continued, subcutaneously at 5000 to 8000 units every 12 hours, during labor and delivery. Low-dose heparin therapy should not alter the aPTT, and laboratory confirmation can be obtained by its measurement on admission. Although these gravidas do not appear to be at any increased risk of postpartum hemorrhage or intraoperative bleeding, the patient's blood type and alloantibody status should be determined by the blood bank during the intrapartum course.

Gravidas with a recent history of a thromboembolic event and those requiring *therapeutic* levels of heparin present a more challenging intrapartum management dilemma. Full-dose heparin, whether administered intravenously or by the subcutaneous route, may be continued throughout labor and stopped just prior to delivery. Alternatively, the patient can be converted to receive an intravenous heparin infusion, which can be stopped 4 hours prior to anticipated delivery to allow the heparin level to slowly decrease. For patients receiving subcutaneous heparin, one method of estimating the hourly intravenous heparin dose is to divide the total daily subcutaneous dose by 24, and begin the hourly infusion at this rate. Subsequent adjustments are made based on the aPTT, measured every 6 hours. However, it may be difficult, particularly in multiparous patients, to accurately estimate the actual time of delivery. A third option includes placing the patient on prophylactic heparin (5000–8000 units every 8–12 hours) during the intrapartum period and resuming full-dose heparin therapy 4 to 6 hours postpartum.

In the event a patient receiving *therapeutic* heparin requires *surgical* intervention or receives an excessive dose of heparin, reversal of the anticoagulant effect can be achieved with protamine sulfate. Administration of 1 mg of protamine will neutralize 100 units of heparin approximately 5 minutes after intravenous administration. The amount of protamine sulfate required can be calculated by direct measurement of the plasma heparin concentration. Unfortunately, the heparin assay required for this calculation is not readily available at most institutions. Thus, the amount of protamine required can be empirically titrated, based on the amount and route of heparin administered, the aPTT, and the half-life of heparin (1–3 hours). It is important not to overestimate the amount of protamine required, as excessive doses have a paradoxical anticoagulant effect. No single dose should exceed 50 mg, and the protamine should be injected over a 10-minute period to prevent hypotension and anaphylaxis.

If a patient has required antepartum anticoagulation with coumarin, fresh frozen plasma can reverse the effect of this long-acting agent. If operative intervention is anticipated, 5 to 10 mg of intramuscular vitamin K will also reverse the coumarin effect. However, 12 hours is required to achieve the optimal effect of a vitamin K injection. The effect of coumarin on the coagulation system can be monitored by the prothrombin time (PT).

Following delivery, patients maintained on low-dose heparin during the antepartum period should be restarted on their prior regimen. Patients at high risk of thromboembolism should have intravenous heparin resumed within 4 to 6 hours of delivery, provided no hemorrhagic complications occurred. Subcutaneous heparin or an oral anticoagulant, regardless of breast-feeding status (22), can then be initiated once the patient reaches a therapeutic level. The hypercoagulable state of pregnancy has been shown to persist as long as 6 weeks following delivery; thus prophylactic or full-dose anticoagulation should be continued throughout this period with serial aPTT or PT measurements as indicated. Careful attention should be directed to ensuring adequate hemostasis at the time of delivery, and surgical wounds should be routinely evaluated for postpartum hematoma.

■ THROMBOCYTOPENIA

Thrombocytopenia is the most commonly encountered platelet abnormality during pregnancy, typically defined as a platelet count less than $150,000/mm^3$. Ideally, the patient with thrombocytopenia will have undergone a complete diagnostic evaluation prior to the onset of labor, allowing optimal management of both mother and fetus. The antenatal evaluation of thrombocytopenia should begin with a thorough history and physical examination. It is important to question a patient carefully regarding recent medication use, as a variety of agents may be responsible for causing the low platelet count (Table 7.7). The initial diagnostic step is to obtain a peripheral blood smear and document the absence of platelet clumping as the cause of a falsely low count.

Table 7.7 *Medications implicated in thrombocytopenia*

Methyldopa

Sedatives

Aspirin

Anticonvulsants

Thiazide diuretics

Sulfa drugs

Ethanol

Estrogens

Quinidine/quinine

Myelosuppressive drugs (e.g. cyclophosphamide)

Additional laboratory studies should be performed (Table 7.8) to exclude decreased bone marrow production, increased peripheral destruction, and abnormal distribution secondary to hypersplenism.

Incidental Thrombocytopenia

With the introduction of automated cell counters into laboratory medicine, asymptomatic thrombocytopenia during pregnancy is now a well-described entity. The incidence of a platelet count lower than 150,000/mm^3 in healthy gravidas with a term gestation has been reported to be 4.6 to 7.6% (23–25). Prenatal investigation of a patient with newly diagnosed thrombocytopenia should ensure an adequate diagnostic evaluation as outlined above. In the absence of an identifiable disease, no specific pharmacologic therapy is indicated for incidental thrombocytopenia of a mild degree.

Table 7.8 *Laboratory evaluation of the thrombocytopenic gravida*

Hematologic

   Complete blood cell count

   Peripheral blood smear

   Bone marrow aspiration

   Red blood cell folate level

   Serum vitamin B_{12} level

Preeclampsia

   Urine protein

   Alanine aminotransferase (ALT)

   Aspartate aminotransferase (AST)

Autoimmune

   Antinuclear antibody (ANA)

   Antiplatelet antibody (PLA-1)

   Lupus anticoagulant (LAC)

   Anticardiolipin antibody

Coagulation

   Prothrombin time (PT)

   Partial thromboplastin time (PTT)

   Fibrinogen

Infectious

   Enzyme-linked immunosorbent assay (ELISA) for HIV
      antibody

Intrapartum considerations include assurance of both maternal and fetal well-being. Available studies suggested that vaginal delivery is acceptable, without further therapy, for asymptomatic patients who have a platelet count above 80,000/mm^3 (26,27). For patients with counts below this relatively arbitrary level, attempts to augment platelet count should be based on associated clinical findings in the individual patient. Epidural anesthesia also has been reported to be safe in parturients with a platelet count above 80,000/mm^3 (24,28). Since the risk of fetal hemorrhage is exceedingly low, determination of fetal platelet count by scalp sampling or cordocentesis is not necessary in patients with incidental thrombocytopenia. Following delivery, serial maternal and fetal platelet counts should be determined to document their stability.

Immune Thrombocytopenic Purpura

Immune thrombocytopenic purpura (ITP) is a disorder of platelet destruction characterized by a platelet count less than 100,000/mm^3 (some would consider < 150,000/mm^3 the lower limit of normal), shortened platelet survival time, and increased megakaryocytes in the bone marrow due to antiplatelet antibodies. The clinical presentation may be acute with sudden-onset bleeding or purpura, or insidious with a long history of easy bruising or recurrent hemorrhage. However, most pregnant patients with ITP are asymptomatic, have only mild to moderate thrombocytopenia, and do not require treatment.

A maternal platelet count below 50,000/mm^3 and active bleeding, regardless of platelet count, are considered indications for instituting medical therapy. Corti-costeroids are currently the treatment of choice and appear to increase the platelet count through bone mar-row stimulation. Intravenous immunoglobulin may be administered to patients who do not respond to a 4- to 6-week trial of steroid therapy. Although ideally avoided during pregnancy, splenectomy may be performed in patients with ITP refractory to medical management. Platelets can be administered acutely for active bleeding, but this is only a temporizing, and often futile, measure since the transfused platelets are rapidly destroyed.

Patients with ITP produce antibody to platelet sur-face antigens, resulting in platelet sequestration and destruction by the reticuloendothelial system. Since most of these antibodies are of the IgG class, they cross the placental barrier and result in fetal platelet destruction and thrombocytopenia. The most significant risk to the fetus is intracranial hemorrhage, usually associated with a fetal platelet count below $50,000/mm^3$. Proponents of the use of cesarean delivery cite the trauma of passage through the birth canal as a major risk for intracranial hemorrhage in thrombocytopenic infants, and advocate that a cesarean section reduces or avoids this risk. How-ever, recommendations in the literature vary widely and do not universally support this position (29–31).

Thus, the most controversial issue in the manage-ment of patients with ITP is estimating the fetal risk of thrombocytopenia and determining the optimal mode of delivery. Unfortunately, maternal platelet count, anti-platelet antibody titers, and platelet-associated IgG do not reliably predict which fetus will be thrombocytope-nic (32–35). Samuels et al (36) reported that the absence of a history of ITP predating pregnancy or the lack of circulating antiplatelet antibody is associated with minimal risk of severe neonatal thrombocytopenia. In contrast, women with a history of ITP had a 20% chance of delivering an infant with severe thrombocytopenia, this occurring only in those patients with circulating antibodies (36). In some centers, absence of both these risk factors is utilized as a criterion for allowing vaginal delivery.

Fetal scalp sampling was the first technique used to determine the fetal platelet count (37). For those who currently advocate scalp sampling in patients with ITP, labor is allowed to continue provided the fetal platelet count is higher than 50,000/mm^3. One of the greatest disadvantages with this method is the need to delay sampling until adequate cervical dilation has been achieved, by which time fetal intracranial hemorrhage could have theoretically occurred. In addition, the platelet count may be falsely lowered due to contamination with amniotic fluid or serous fluid of the scalp. Although the number of patients studied was small, Christiaens and Helmerhorst (38) demonstrated that nearly half of intrapartum fetal scalp samples had a falsely low platelet count. Furthermore, observing a clot in the scalp sample does not guarantee a normal fetal platelet count (39). Based on these latter issues, this intrapartum approach to predicting subsequent neonatal hemorrhage has been questioned.

Cordocentesis has also been utilized to sample fetal blood from patients with ITP (40–42). When the patient at risk for neonatal thrombocytopenia undergoes cordocentesis at 37 weeks' gestation or later, a trial of labor is recommended if the fetal platelet count is more than

50,000/mm^3. This procedure offers the advantage of being performed electively prior to the onset of labor and engagement of the fetal head. Cordocentesis has the additional benefit of allowing both fetuses to be sampled in a twin pregnancy affected by ITP. However, given the limited number of cases studied, the hemorrhagic risk of the procedure in a severely thrombocytopenic fetus is unclear. Opponents argue that the risk of the procedure is unjustified given the overall low incidence of severe fetal thrombocytopenia and hemorrhage. The role of cordocentesis in the management of patients with ITP remains controversial and investigation continues.

The optimal approach to predicting neonatal hemorrhage in the face of maternal ITP has not been established. Thus, clinicians use various combinations of the above-mentioned strategies in the management of these patients. Once a delivery plan has been formulated, the maternal platelet count should be determined at admission. In women who have received steroid therapy within the previous 4 weeks, 100 mg of intravenous hydrocortisone should be administered every 8 hours during labor and 24 hours following delivery, to prevent an adrenal crisis. Placement of a fetal scalp electrode, pH determination, and operative vaginal delivery should be avoided unless the fetal platelet count is known and above 100,000/mm^3. Consultation with an anesthesiologist prior to the onset of active labor to determine if the individual patient is a candidate for regional anesthesia is prudent. Intravenous narcotics may be administered as indicated for pain relief.

Patients with ITP do not appear to be at significantly increased risk of postpartum hemorrhage when the maternal platelet count is higher than $100,000/mm^3$. However, the incidence has been reported to increase from 4 to 33% when the platelet count falls below this level (43). Heys (44) observed that episiotomy sites and areas of perineal trauma were the most common sources of postpartum hemorrhage in patients with ITP. Thus, careful examination and repair of the perineum should be performed.

Intrapartum platelet transfusion is not warranted unless operative delivery is required with a platelet count lower than $50,000/mm^3$ or in the presence of active bleeding. In the event a surgical procedure is performed with platelets at this level, 10 units of platelet concentrate may be administered immediately prior to making the incision. If no hemorrhagic complications are encountered intraoperatively, additional units of platelets should not be infused. The life span of transfused platelets is exceedingly short in ITP, given the presence of circulating antibodies. The risk of additional platelet transfusion is unwarranted in the stable patient.

■ **REFERENCES**

1. Newton M, Mosey LM, Egli GE, Gifford WB, Hull CT. Blood loss during and immediately after delivery. Obstet Gynecol 1961;17:9.
2. Pritchard JA, Baldwin RM, Dickey JC, et al. Blood volume changes in pregnancy and the puerperium. II. Red blood cell loss and changes in apparent blood volume during and following vaginal delivery, cesarean section, and cesarean section plus total hysterectomy. Am J Obstet Gynecol 1962;84:1271.

3. Blattner P, Dar H, Nitowski HM. Pregnancy outcome in women with sickle cell trait. JAMA 1977;238:1392.

4. Whalley PJ, Martin FG, Pritchard JA. Sickle cell trait and urinary tract infections during pregnancy. JAMA 1964;189: 903.

5. McColgin SW, Morrison JC. Anemia associated with chronic systemic disorders. In: Gleicher N, ed. Principles and practice of medical therapy in pregnancy. 2nd ed. New York: Appleton & Lange, 1992:1009.

6. Cunningham FG, Pritchard JA, Mason R. Pregnancy and sickle cell hemoglobinopathies: results with and without prophylactic transfusions. Obstet Gynecol 1983;62:419–424.

7. Morrison JC, Schneider JM, Whybrew WD, Bucovaz ET, Menzel DM. Prophylactic transfusions in pregnant patients with sickle hemoglobinopathies: benefit versus risk. Obstet Gynecol 1980;56:274–280.

8. Koshy M, Burd L, Wallace D, Moawad A, Baron J. Prophylactic red-cell transfusions in pregnant patients with sickle cell disease. A randomized cooperative study. N Engl J Med 1988;319:1447–1452.

9. Charache S, Niebyl JR. Pregnancy in sickle cell disease. Clin Hematol 1985;14:729.

10. Charache S, Scott J, Niebyl J, Bonds D. Management of sickle cell disease in pregnant patients. Obstet Gynecol 1980;55:407.

11. Bassell GM, Horbelt DV. Hematologic disease. In: Datta S, ed. Anesthetic and obstetric management of high-risk pregnancy. St. Louis: Mosby Year Book, 1991:345.

12. Laros RK Jr. Maternal hematologic disorders. In: Creasy RK, Resnick R, eds. Maternal-fetal medicine: principles and practice. 3rd ed. Philadelphia: WB Saunders Company, 1994:905.

13. McVay PA, Hoag RW, Hoag MS, Toy PTCY. Safety and use of autologous blood donation during the third tri-

mester of pregnancy. Am J Obstet Gynecol 1989;160: 1479–1488.

14. Herbert WNP, Owen HG, Collins ML. Autologous blood storage in obstetrics. Obstet Gynecol 1988;72:166–170.

15. Andres RL, Piacquadio KM, Resnik R. A reappraisal of the need for autologous blood donation in the obstetric patient. Am J Obstet Gynecol 1990;163:1551–1553.

16. Combs CA, Murphy EL, Laros RK. Cost-benefit analysis of autologous blood donation in obstetrics. Obstet Gynecol 1992;80:621–625.

17. Rackow EC, Weil MH. Recent trends in diagnosis and management of septic shock. Curr Probl Surg 1983;40: 181.

18. Development Task Force of the College of American Pathologists. Practice parameters for the use of fresh-frozen plasma, cryoprecipitate, and platelets. JAMA 1994:271: 777–781.

19. Hewitt PE, Machin SJ. Massive blood transfusion. BMJ 1990;300:107.

20. Committee on Standards. Standards for blood banks and transfusion services. 13th ed. Arlington, VA: American Association of Blood Banks, 1989.

21. Boyan CP, Howland WS. Cardiac arrest and temperature of bank blood. JAMA 1963;183:58–60.

22. Committee on Drugs. American Academy of Pediatrics. Transfer of drugs and other chemicals into human milk. Pediatrics 1989;84:924–936.

23. Burrows RF, Kelton JG. Incidentally detected thrombocytopenia in healthy mothers and their infants. N Engl J Med 1988;319:142–145.

24. Burrows RF, Kelton JG. Thrombocytopenia at delivery: a prospective survey of 6715 deliveries. Am J Obstet Gynecol 1990;162:731–734.

25. Freedman J, Musclow E, Garvey B, Abbott D. Unex-

plained periparturient thrombocytopenia. Am J Hematol 1986;21:397.

26. Burrows RF, Kelton JG. Thrombocytopenia during pregnancy. In: Greer IA, Turpie AGG, Forbes CD, eds. Haemostasis and thrombosis in obstetrics and gynaecology. London: Chapman and Hall, 1992:407–429.

27. Aster RH. "Gestational" thrombocytopenia: a plea for conservative management. N Engl J Med 1990;323:264–6.

28. Letsky EA. Haemostasis and epidural anaesthesia. Int J Obstet Anesth 1991;1:51–54.

29. Laros RK, Sweet RL. Management of idiopathic thrombocytopenic purpura during pregnancy. Am J Obstet Gynecol 1975;122:182.

30. Laros RK, Kagan R. Route of delivery for patients with immune thrombocytopenic purpura. Am J Obstet Gynecol 1984;148:901.

31. Murray JM, Harris RE. The management of the pregnant patient with idiopathic thrombocytopenic purpura. Am J Obstet Gynecol 1976;126:449.

32. Territo M, Finklestein J, Oh W, Hobel C, Kattlove H. Management of autoimmune thrombocytopenia in pregnancy and the neonate. Obstet Gynecol 1973;41:579.

33. Cines DB, Dusak B, Tomaski A, Mennuti M, Schreiber AD. Immune thrombocytopenic purpura and pregnancy. N Engl J Med 1982;306:826.

34. Kelton JG, Inwood MJ, Barr RM, et al. The prenatal prediction of thrombocytopenia in infants of mothers with clinically diagnosed immune thrombocytopenia. Am J Obstet Gynecol 1982;144:449.

35. Laros RK Jr. Maternal hematologic disorders. In: Creasy RK, Resnick R, eds. Maternal-fetal medicine: principles and practice. 3rd ed. Philadelphia: WB Saunders Company, 1994:476.

36. Samuels P, Bussel JB, Braitman LE, et al. Estimation of the

risk of thrombocytopenia in the offspring of pregnant women with presumed immune thrombocytopenic purpura. N Engl J Med 1990;323:229–235.

37. Ayromlooi J. A new approach to the management of immunologic thrombocytopenic purpura in pregnancy. Am J Obstet Gynecol 1978;130:235.

38. Christiaens GCML, Helmerhorst FM. Validity of intrapartum diagnosis of fetal thrombocytopenia. Am J Obstet Gynecol 1987;157:864–865.

39. Moise KJ Jr, Patton DE, Cano LE. Misdiagnosis of a normal fetal platelet count after coagulation of intrapartum scalp samples in autoimmune thrombocytopenic purpura. Am J Perinatol 1991;8:295–296.

40. Scioscia AL, Grannum PAT, Copel JA, Hobbins JC. The use of percutaneous umbilical blood sampling in immune thrombocytopenic purpura. Am J Obstet Gynecol 1988; 159:1066–1068.

41. Moise KJ, Carpenter RJ, Cotton DB, Wasserstrum N, Kirshon B, Cano L. Percutaneous umbilical cord blood sampling in the evaluation of fetal platelet counts in pregnant patients with autoimmune thrombocytopenia purpura. Obstet Gynecol 1988;72:346–350.

42. Daffos F, Forestier F, Kaplan C, Cox W. Prenatal diagnosis and management of bleeding disorders with fetal blood sampling. Am J Obstet Gynecol 1988;158:939.

43. O'Reilly RA, Taber B. Immunologic thrombocytopenic purpura and pregnancy. Obstet Gynecol 1978;51:590.

44. Heys RF. Child bearing and idiopathic thrombocytopenic purpura. Br J Obstet Gynaecol 1966;73:205.

Neurologic Disease

▼　▼　▼　▼　▼

■ SEIZURE DISORDER

Epilepsy is one of the more common neurologic disorders found in women of reproductive age. The disorder may predate or appear for the first time during gestation, and pregnancy has a variable and unpredictable effect on seizure frequency. Depending on the gestational age and clinical presentation, eclampsia must be included in the differential diagnosis of new-onset seizures. Additional etiologies in a patient who has never had a convulsion include tumor, vascular malformation, infection, electrolyte disturbance, and substance abuse or withdrawal. Although it is usually not possible to predict the disease course in any given pregnant woman with preexisting epilepsy, the occurrence of seizures remains unchanged in approximately 50%, increases in 25%, and decreases in 25% of patients (1).

Various medications are employed for seizure control, and ideally a patient's regimen should be optimized prior to pregnancy. Although all antiseizure preparations have been implicated in teratogenesis, most often the benefits of treatment outweigh the risks. Due to the physiologic alterations of pregnancy, including decreased gastrointestinal absorption and protein binding, and increased plasma volume and renal clearance, serum anticonvulsant levels may decrease throughout pregnancy. Therefore, frequent monitoring of drug levels and adjustments in dosing may be required to maintain a therapeutic concentration of an individual agent. Consultation with a neurologist during the antepartum period will facilitate comprehensive care of the patient.

Although postpartum hemorrhage, cesarean delivery, and low-birth-weight infants reportedly occur at a higher rate (2,3), it does not appear that women with epilepsy are at an increased risk of preeclampsia, abruptio placentae, or premature delivery (4). The most significant threat to the patient and the fetus is an intrapartum seizure, as this can result in maternal trauma and fetal hypoxia and death. When labor commences in a patient with a seizure disorder, a careful evaluation of her antiseizure medication regimen, recent serum levels, and compliance is essential. Because a subtherapeutic drug concentration is associated with an increased risk of convulsion, patients should continue to receive their antiseizure agents during labor. Oral medications can be continued with a sip of water, but the parenteral form may be considered given the decreased intestinal absorption that occurs during labor (Table 8.1). The plasma drug concentration of anticonvulsants should be monitored closely following delivery as medication requirements may decrease by 50% in the initial postpartum period.

Adequate analgesia may decrease patient anxiety, hyperventilation, and the associated respiratory alkalosis that can exacerbate a seizure. It is important to be aware of the interactions between anticonvulsant medications and systemic analgesics and anesthetic agents. For

Table 8.1 Commonly used anticonvulsants oral and parenteral dosing

Medication	Oral Dose	Equivalent parenteral dose	Therapeutic serum level
Phenytoin	100–300 mg tid	1 mg PO = 1 mg IV	10–20 μg/mL
Phenobarbital	100–200 mg tid–qid	4–6 mg/kg/day in 3 divided doses	10–40 μg/mL
Carbamazepine	200 mg bid–qid	Not available	4–8 μg/mL
Valproic acid	15–60 mg/kg/day	Not available	50–100 μg/mL

instance, women taking phenobarbital may have an increased or decreased requirement for opiates, depending on the duration the barbiturate has been taken. Phenytoin may be associated with hepatitis, liver dysfunction, and decreased clearance of anesthetics. Although it is unclear whether spinal anesthesia exacerbates epilepsy, epidural anesthesia has been used without evidence of adverse effects on seizure frequency (5).

Patients with well-controlled seizures do not require induction of labor providing there are no complicating medical or obstetric factors. Most women can expect a normal vaginal delivery (4), and cesarean section should be reserved for standard obstetric indications. Although data are lacking, it has been empirically suggested that elective cesarean delivery be considered in patients with substantial neurologic or mental deficit, very poor seizure control late in pregnancy, or a prior occurrence of severe seizures associated with significant physical or emotional stress (6). An emergent cesarean section may be required for fetal indications following a grand mal seizure. However, maternal stabilization prior to operative intervention is essential to prevent further complications in a woman who has just had a seizure. As with eclampsia, in utero resuscitation of the transiently hypoxic fetus is the preferential approach prior to considering operative delivery.

A grand mal seizure occurs during labor in 1 to 2% of women with epilepsy, and an additional 1 to 2% of patients experience a convulsion during the postpartum period (6). Whenever a patient has a seizure, all attempts must be made to determine the underlying etiology. As mentioned, an evaluation for eclampsia should be undertaken depending on other clinical factors, such as gestational age. A careful history should include questions regarding recent sleep deprivation, symptoms of infection, and noncompliance with medication. Laboratory evaluation should include a drug level to determine the need for dosage adjustments. If a seizure is different in nature from the patient's previous seizures, an extensive evaluation is indicated to exclude a new focal deficit. Consultation with a neurologist will aid the clinician in obtaining appropriate testing.

A patient who has a new-onset seizure requires a more thorough evaluation than a patient with recurrent convulsions. Laboratory evaluation should include a hemoglobin measurement, white blood cell and platelet counts, and a urine drug screening. A metabolic aberration should be excluded by measuring serum electrolytes, urea, creatinine, glucose, magnesium, calcium, and phosphorus. Computed tomography of the head with abdominal shielding will provide information regarding the presence of a stroke or tumor as the inciting factor. The remainder of the evaluation should be guided by additional history and physical examination findings at admission.

Status epilepticus is a state in which seizures occur without full recovery between them or a seizure that has a duration of more than 30 minutes. It occurs in less than 1% of patients with a seizure disorder, but maternal and fetal mortality are significant. Although status may occur with petit mal and focal seizures, generalized tonic-clonic status is the most frequent and life-threatening type. The most important principle is to control the status as quickly as possible because the longer status persists, the more difficult it becomes to interrupt. Complications of status include neuronal damage, hypoxia, acidosis, cardiopulmonary decompensation, rhabdomyolysis, myoglobinuric acute renal failure, hyperthermia, and coagulopathy. Adverse fetal effects are the direct result of maternal hypoxia and alterations in uteroplacental blood flow.

The initial management of an intrapartum patient in status epilepticus includes airway maintenance, oxygen administration, establishment of intravenous access, and prevention of injury (Table 8.2). Laboratory studies should be performed, recognizing that empiric therapy is necessary prior to the availability of these results. Intravenous thiamine is administered in the event that

Table 8.2 *Management of status epilepticus*

Blood sample for:

    Electrolytes, urea, glucose, creatinine, calcium, magnesium, and phosphorus

    Anticonvulsant levels

    Toxicity screen (e.g., alcohol, cocaine)

    Arterial blood gas

Thiamine (100 mg in first liter of intravenous normal saline solution)

Intravenous bolus of 1 ampule 50% dextrose solution

Diazepam (2 mg/min intravenously until seizures stop or a total of 20 mg)

Initiate anticonvulsant therapy (e.g., phenytoin) for control of subsequent seizure activity

---

the seizure was precipitated by a deficiency of this vitamin, and dextrose solution is given to correct for the
possibility of profound hypoglycemia. Although bolus
diazepam will stop seizures, it does not prevent further
activity. Diazepam has been noted to decrease fetal heart
rate variability, with newborn effects being most notable
at doses larger than 30 mg (7,8).

An anticonvulsant agent must be administered in a
timely fashion for continued seizure control. Phenytoin
is the preferred agent as it has less respiratory depression and alteration of consciousness compared to phenobarbital. Based on clinical experience with phenytoin
prophylaxis in preeclampsia, Ryan et al (9) suggested
dividing the loading dose into an initial bolus of 10 mg/
kg (pregnant weight) followed by 5 mg/kg in 2 hours.
Maintenance therapy is then begun 12 hours after the
loading dose is completed. This dosing regimen (Table
8.3) results in a therapeutic serum level with minimal

Table 8.3 *Suggested protocol for phenytoin administration**

Dose	15 mg/kg (pregnant weight)
Administer	10 mg/kg bolus
	5 mg/kg 2 hr later
Dilute	Total dose in 100–250 mL of normal saline
Infuse	< 50 mg/min
Flush	Normal saline if burning occurs

*Reprinted by permission from Ryan G, Lange IR, Naugler MA. Clin-
ical experience with phenytoin prophylaxis in severe preeclampsia.
Am J Obstet Gynecol 1989;161:1297–1304.

side effects (9). Infusion of phenytoin should not exceed 50 mg/minute as hypotension may result.

If seizure activity persists despite the phenytoin load, several second-line approaches can be attempted based on the clinician's past experience. This may include the use of intravenous phenobarbital at an infusion ate of less than 100 mg/minute until seizures stop or a total dose of 20 mg/kg is achieved. Alternatively, a continuous intravenous diazepam infusion (501–100 mg of diazepam in 500 mL of dextrose in water at a rate of 40 mL/hr) can be tried. If seizures continue, general anesthesia and endotracheal intubation should be performed.

■ MYASTHENIA GRAVIS

Myasthenia gravis (MG) is an autoimmune neuromuscular disorder characterized by weakness and easy fatigability of skeletal muscles. A patient typically presents with symptoms of weakness of the facial muscles that gradually progress to other muscle groups. The underlying etiology of the disease is an antibody of the IgG class against the nicotinic acetylcholine receptors at the neuromuscular junction. Myasthenia is frequently associated with other autoimmune phenomena including the presence of antithyroid and antinuclear antibodies and rheumatoid factor. The diagnosis is established by the injection of edrophonium chloride followed by documentation of the reversal of muscle weakness. Electrophysiologic testing also may be employed to quantify the neuromuscular deficit.

The maternal risks associated with myasthenia in pregnancy include exacerbation of disease, myasthenic crisis, adverse drug reactions, respiratory failure, and death. Pregnancy may affect the course of the disease, improving in one third of patients, showing worsening symptoms in one third, and remaining stable in a third (10). It has been postulated that the increased rate of premature delivery is related to the oxytocic effects of acetylcholinesterase inhibitors. Transient neonatal MG is secondary to the transplacental passage of antibodies to the acetylcholine receptors and occurs in approximately 15% of neonates.

The first-line treatment of MG is with quaternary ammonium compounds that inhibit the destruction of acetylcholine at the myoneural junction. Pyridostigmine is the most commonly used agent because it has a longer duration of action than other drugs of this class. Measurements of grip strength or vital capacity have been used to follow the drug's efficacy during the antenatal period. Additionally, corticosteroids may be administered to control the disease and are particularly effective in young women. Although not all are applicable during pregnancy, other treatment regimens have included azathioprine, gamma globulins, plasmapheresis, and thymectomy.

It is important to carefully monitor medications that are administered to a patient with MG during labor. The oral anticholinesterase medication should be administered via the intramuscular or intravenous route as gastrointestinal absorption may be unpredictable with the onset of labor. Parenteral pyridostigmine is administered at one thirtieth of the patient's oral dose. The intravenous preparation must be given slowly and the patient carefully observed for signs of a cholinergic reaction (abdominal cramps, nausea, vomiting, diarrhea, miosis, increased salivation and bronchial secretions, diaphoresis). Of note, muscle weakness may be a sign of either undertreatment or overtreatment of myasthenia. A patient who has received steroid therapy within the previous 4 weeks should be treated with hydrocortisone (100 mg given intravenously every 8 hours) to prevent an adrenal crisis. Magnesium sulfate is contraindicated as it diminishes the depolarizing action of acetylcholine, worsens muscle weakness, and may precipitate a myasthenic crisis. Therefore, patients with preeclampsia should be given an alternative antiseizure medication. Patients with MG also appear to be more susceptible to the depressant effects of narcotics, barbiturates, tranquilizers, and volatile anesthetics, and these should be used judiciously. Antibiotic regimens should also be chosen carefully so as to avoid agents that may worsen the patient's symptoms. Table 8.4 lists specific medications that should be avoided in patients with MG.

Since the uterus contains smooth muscle that is unaffected by the disease process, the first stage of labor should progress normally in the myasthenic patient. However, skeletal muscle weakness may result in decreased maternal expulsive forces during the second stage of labor, and forceps- or vacuum-assisted delivery may be required. Cesarean section should be reserved for standard obstetric indications. Use of a regional anesthetic during labor and delivery provides excellent pain relief and eliminates the need for intravenous analgesics, which may depress respiratory function.

The stress of labor and delivery may precipitate a myasthenic crisis during the intrapartum and postpartum periods. Other associated factors include infection, a surgical procedure, and a change in the patient's anticholinergic medication. A crisis is characterized by an acute exacerbation of myasthenic symptoms resulting in the need for mechanical ventilation. Therefore, the patient's respiratory status should be carefully monitored for signs of fatigue and the resultant hypoxia. Serial vital capacity measurements may be performed if there is any suspicion of respiratory compromise. Early consultation with a neurologist familiar with the patient's condition is recommended in these circumstances.

■ SPINAL CORD INJURY

Spinal cord transection resulting in paraplegia or quadriplegia is most commonly caused by trauma. Infection,

Table 8.4 *Medications that adversely affect patients with myasthenia gravis*

Narcotics
Tranquilizers
Barbiturates
Inhalation anesthetics
Ether
Halothane
Trichlorethylene
Magnesium salts
Lithium
Penicillamine
Beta-adrenergic agents
Quinidine
Aminoglycosides

tumor, or a vascular lesion may also result in permanent spinal cord damage. Advances in acute care and rehabilitation of patients with a spinal cord injury have allowed more young women to reach a point of desiring pregnancy and childbirth. Although a normal menstrual cycle may be acutely interrupted following the injury, fertility does not appear to be adversely affected. These patients are at an increased risk of decubitus ulcers, urinary tract infection, autonomic hyperreflexia (see below), deep venous thrombosis, and pulmonary complications. Depending on the level of the lesion, pregnant women may be unable to perceive contractions, thus increasing the risk of preterm and unattended births.

Labor may progress normally through the first stage because uterine smooth muscle is unaffected by the patient's spinal cord injury. Maternal expulsive forces may be compromised, and operative vaginal delivery is commonly performed to facilitate the second stage of labor. Cesarean section should be reserved for obstetric indications or when there is intractable hyperreflexia despite optimal treatment. Although anesthesia is often not required for pain control, autonomic hyperreflexia can be prevented by placement of epidural anesthesia to a level of T10. Combinations of low concentrations of local anesthetics and narcotics through the epidural route are effective in blocking noxious sensory input, thus blunting the uncontrolled sympathetic reflex. A single-injection spinal block can be equally effective, although the anesthetic spread is somewhat unpredictable and the duration of action is limited. Anesthetic-induced hypotension should be avoided through adequate prehydration and uterine displacement.

Ephedrine in its usual dosage (5–15 mg intravenously) can be safely used in the spinal cord injury patient to correct transient hypotension.

Autonomic hyperreflexia can be life threatening and represents the most significant intrapartum risk. Hyperreflexia may be activated by almost any cutaneous or visceral stimuli below the lesion, including pelvic examination, uterine contractions, and bowel or bladder distention. This reflex results from a sudden, uninhibited sympathetic discharge below the level of paralysis for which the parasympathetic system cannot compensate. Patients with lesions above the upper thoracic segments are most susceptible to this reflex as the major sympathetic outflow occurs between T5 and L2. The syndrome has occurred in 66 to 85% of patients with an injury above T7 (11). Patients experience a sudden onset of anxiety, sweating, headache, and increased muscle twitching. Objective signs include severe hypertension, skin blotching, a reactive sinus bradycardia, and cardiac arrhythmias.

When autonomic hyperreflexia occurs, it is crucial to rapidly remove the precipitating stimulus. Elevation of the head of the patient's bed is a quick, initial maneuver that may have some antihypertensive effect. Severe hypertension should be treated aggressively because uncontrolled hypertension can result in retinal, cerebral, or subarachnoid hemorrhage (SAH) and subsequent convulsions. Treatment options include hydralazine, labetalol, trimethaphan, nitroprusside, and nitroglycerin (see Table 1.5). Placement of epidural anesthesia has been advocated as one of the more effective options available for the treatment of autonomic hyperreflexia (12).

During the postpartum period, patients should be properly assisted in resuming their usual self-care regimens. Close attention should be given to reducing the development of pressure ulcers. An increased frequency of episiotomy dehiscence was reported in two small series of patients with spinal cord injuries (13,14). Although no data are available, the patient's immobility combined with the hypercoagulable state of pregnancy suggests that heparin prophylaxis against venous thrombosis may be of benefit. Postpartum respiratory and physical therapy may also aid the patient during recovery from an operative delivery.

■ MULTIPLE SCLEROSIS

Multiple sclerosis (MS) is a demyelinating disease that takes one of two forms: relapsing-remitting disease with multiple nervous system lesions, or chronic disease with progressive spinal cord dysfunction. It occurs most frequently in women 20 to 40 years old. Patients commonly experience bladder disturbances, sensory symptoms, diplopia, and speech and gait difficulties. Frequent physical findings include optic disk pallor, cerebellar ataxia, dysarthria, hyperreflexia, spasticity, and weakness of the lower extremities. The course and severity of this disease vary between individuals but it is characterized by exacerbations and remissions.

Treatment is primarily supportive during periods of remission. Corticosteroids are generally administered only during an acute exacerbation or with rapidly progressive disease. Baclofen and dantrolene have been used to treat painful flexor or extensor spasms of the lower extremities. Patients with bladder dysfunction are at higher risk for the development of urinary tract infection, particularly in the presence of a gravid uterus.

MS does not appear to affect the course of labor and delivery. The degree of difficulty encountered intrapartum by the patient with MS depends on the disease stage and neurologic deficits present. A patient with uncomplicated disease can expect a course of labor similar to that of women without MS. The patient who has more significant disease manifestations such as severe spasticity may have difficulty during the second stage of labor. Baclofen may be administered intrapartum to patients who experience these spasms, and the optimal dosage for control of the patient's symptoms requires individual titration. Therefore, medication taken during the antepartum period may be used as a guide to facilitate dosing. Otherwise, the initial dose is 5 mg orally three times daily, and can be increased to a maximum of 80 mg/day. If steroid therapy was administered within the previous 4 weeks for an exacerbation, 100 mg of intravenous hydrocortisone should be given every 8 hours during labor and for 24 hours postpartum. Although there are limited data on the effects of conduction anesthesia in patients with MS, there is no evidence to contraindicate its use. Epidural anesthesia during labor may have the additional advantage of decreasing abdominal and pelvic muscle spasticity, which can interfere with spontaneous delivery. Patients should be carefully observed during the initial 3 months postpartum as it appears that the highest frequency of exacerbation is observed during this time.

■ INTRACRANIAL HEMORRHAGE

Intracranial hemorrhage (ICH) is a life-threatening complication that can occur in the pregnant population. The major cause of ICH in pregnancy is SAH from a cerebral aneurysm or arteriovenous malformation (AVM) rupture. The incidence of SAH in the pregnant population is 1 in 10,000, with a reported immediate mortality rate of 43% (15). Pregnancy-induced hypertension is associated with intracerebral pathology, including ICH, which may account for up to 60% of the deaths associated with eclampsia. Less common etiologies for ICH include dural venous sinus thrombosis, mycotic aneurysm, choriocarcinoma, vasculitides, and coagulopathies. Recently, cocaine and phenylpropanolamine were associated with ICH in the pregnant patient (16). The remainder of this section focuses on the peripartum management of patients with cerebral aneurysm or AVM. Preeclampsia-related issues are discussed in Chapter 1.

Certain groups of patients are at increased risk of cerebral aneurysm, including those with a family history and those having one of a diverse collection of rare disorders (e.g., polycystic kidney disease, Marfan's syndrome, Ehlers-Danlos syndrome). Most aneurysms and AVMs remain asymptomatic until bleeding occurs, when the patient presents with the complaint of severe headache or demonstrates seizures, focal neurologic signs, or altered consciousness. Patients who have undergone successful surgical correction of either of these lesions prior to delivery do not merit any special intrapartum considerations.

Three major complications can occur in the pregnant

patient suffering from a SAH who survives transport to the hospital: 1) hydrocephalus, 2) vasospasm, and 3) rebleed. Hydrocephalus may occur at any time in the first 2 weeks following SAH. The chief danger of hydrocephalus is compression of the brain stem, leading to a progressive deterioration in the level of consciousness and respiratory function. The treatment of this complication is drainage of the cerebrospinal fluid through a ventriculostomy. Vasospasm following SAH can lead to cerebral ischemia and seizures. The treatment for vasospasm remains controversial, and includes the use of volume expansion, induced hypertension, and calcium entry blockers. Recurrent bleeds are associated with a much higher mortality rate than that seen with the initial bleeding episode. Aneurysms tend to rebleed at 7 to 10 days, whereas subsequent bleeding with AVMs is infrequent and late. During pregnancy, an accessible lesion should be repaired to prevent the high incidence of significant morbidity and mortality associated with a recurrent bleed.

Most data pertaining to the intrapartum management of ruptured cerebral aneurysms and AVMs are anecdotally derived. In the nonlaboring patient, maternal stabilization and spontaneous onset of labor are advocated. However, during the labor process, the most frequent obstetric concern relates to the mode of delivery. Although previous literature suggested elective cesarean section for cerebral aneurysm patients, more recent data support vaginal delivery in that this approach poses no additional risk to the mother and fetus (17). Young et al (18) proposed that during contractions, intracranial transvessel gradients remain static, thereby supporting the above-mentioned clinical recommendations. Conversely, most clinicians would attempt to minimize second-stage Valsalva maneuvering by performing early operative vaginal delivery. The intrapartum management of the patient with an AVM is less clear as there is the suggestion that these vessels are more liable to rebleed during labor. Therefore, some authorities advocate elective cesarean delivery, while others allow vaginal delivery (17,19,20). Conduction anesthesia has been recommended for labor and delivery management for both cerebral aneurysm and AVM (17,21).

In the moribund ICH patient with a fetus at a viable gestational age, ethical considerations mandate individualized decision making. Appropriate timing of delivery should be based on the institution's ability to care for the premature neonate. Evidence for a preferred route of delivery is lacking, with no clear contraindication to vaginal delivery.

■ REFERENCES

1. Patterson RM. Seizure disorders in pregnancy. Med Clin North Am 1989;73:661–665.
2. Bjerkedal T, Bahna SL. The course and outcome of pregnancy in women with epilepsy. Acta Obstet Gynecol Scand 1973;52:245.
3. Yerby MS, Koepsell T, Daling J. Pregnancy complications and outcomes in a cohort of women with epilepsy. Epilepsia 1985;26:631–635.
4. Hiilesmaa VK, Bardy A, Teramo K. Obstetric outcome in women with epilepsy. Am J Obstet Gynecol 1985;152:499–504.
5. Santos AC, Petrikovsky BM, Kaplan GP. Neurologic and muscular diseases. In: Datta S, ed. Anesthetic and obstet-

ric management of high-risk pregnancy. St. Louis: Mosby Year Book, 1991:35–68.

6. Hiilesmaa VK. Pregnancy and birth in women with epilepsy. Neurology 1992(suppl 5);42:8–11.

7. Yeh SY, Paul RH, Cordero L, Hon EH. A study of diazepam during labor. Obstet Gynecol 1974;43:363–373.

8. Cree JE, Meyer J, Hailey DM. Diazepam in labour: its metabolism and effect on the clinical condition and thermogenesis of the newborn. BMJ 1973;4:251–255.

9. Ryan G, Lange IR, Naugler MA. Clinical experience with phenytoin prophylaxis in severe preeclampsia. Am J Obstet Gynecol 1989;161:1297–1304.

10. Plauche WC. Myasthenia gravis in pregnancy: an update. Am J Obstet Gynecol 1979;135:691–697.

11. McGregor JA, Meeurosen J. Autonomic hyperreflexia: a mortal danger for spinal cord-damaged women in labor. Am J Obstet Gynecol 1985;151:330.

12. Wanner MB, Rageth CJ, Zach GA. Pregnancy and autonomic hyperreflexia in patients with spinal cord lesions. Paraplegia 1987;25:482–490.

13. Werduyn WH. Spinal cord injured women, pregnancy and delivery. Paraplegia 1986;24:231–240.

14. Hughes SJ, Short DJ, Usherwood MM, Tebbutt H. Management of the pregnant woman with spinal cord injuries. Br J Obstet Gynaecol 1991;98:513–518.

15. Pakarinen S. Incidence, aetiology, and prognosis of primary subarachnoid hemorrhage. Acta Neurol Scand 1967; 43:128.

16. Henderson CE, Torbey M. Rupture of intracranial aneurysm associated with cocaine use during pregnancy. Am J Perinatol 1988;5:142–143.

17. Dias MS, Sekhar LN. Intracranial hemorrhage from aneurysms and arteriovenous malformations during pregnancy and the puerperium. Neurosurgery 1990;27:855–866.

18. Young DC, Leveno KJ, Walley PS. Induced delivery prior to surgery for ruptured cerebral aneurysm. Obstet Gynecol 1983;53:285–288.

19. Weibers DO. Subarachnoid hemorrhage in pregnancy. Semin Neurol 1988;8:226–229.

20. Dalessio DJ. Neurologic diseases. In: Burrow GN, Ferris TF, eds. Medical complications during pregnancy. 2nd ed. Philadelphia: WB Saunders Company, 1982:435–447.

21. Hunt HB, Schifrin BS, Suzuki K. Ruptured berry aneurysms and pregnancy. Obstet Gynecol 1974;43:827–837.

Critical Care Obstetrics

▼   ▼   ▼   ▼   ▼

■ MONITORING TECHNIQUES

Pulse Oximetry

Pulse oximetry has become one of the more commonly utilized noninvasive monitoring devices in clinical medicine. It is an alternative to arterial blood gas sampling and provides continuous information regarding oxygenation. Studies of this device in pregnancy demonstrated its usefulness during labor and cesarean delivery (1).

The oximeter consists of a sensor containing a light-emitting diode and a photodetector. This sensor measures changes in the transmission of alternating beams of red and infrared light that pass through a pulsatile vascular bed. Oxyhemoglobin and deoxyhemoglobin have fixed patterns of absorbance. The pulse oximeter correlates these patterns to determine the amount of saturated hemoglobin, expressed as a percentage of total hemoglobin present.

The normal oxygen saturation reported by a pulse oximeter during pregnancy is 96 to 100%. Although the oximeter accurately reflects oxygenation, it is important to recognize that the saturation will not be less than 95% until the partial pressure of oxygen (PO_2) has fallen below 60 mm Hg (Figure 9.1). Thus, in the critically ill

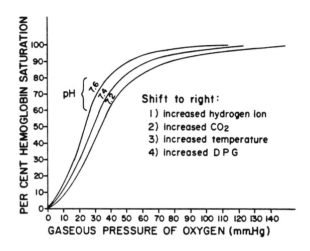

Fig. 9.1 *Oxygen dissociation curve.*

patient with an oximetry saturation less than 95%, an arterial blood gas sample should be obtained to more accurately determine the level of hypoxemia.

Arterial Line

Accurate information regarding arterial blood pressure is important in caring for critically ill patients. In spite of various noninvasive methods, an arterial catheter permits the most precise determination of blood pressure on a continuous basis. Additionally, patients with evidence of respiratory compromise who require serial blood gas assessment often benefit from the placement of an arterial catheter because it decreases the vessel trauma and discomfort associated with obtaining multiple arterial samples. Patients who are in shock, are hypotensive, or require vasoactive agents for blood pressure support or control (e.g., dopamine or sodium nitro-prusside, respectively) are candidates for an arterial line.

Mean arterial pressure (MAP) and pulse pressure are two parameters derived from the systolic (SBP) and diastolic (DBP) blood pressures. Mean arterial pressure may be approximated (MAP = DBP + $^1/_3$ [SBP–DBP]), calculated by an electronic blood pressure device, or measured directly via an arterial line. Mean arterial pressure is the average pressure in the aorta and its major branches during a particular cardiac cycle, and is dependent on cardiac output and peripheral resistance. Pulse pressure is the difference between SBP and DBP and corresponds to a change in intravascular volume. As such, in the setting of obstetric hemorrhage, pulse pressure may be more helpful than SBP or DBP alone. Decreased pulse pressure is often an initial sign of hypovolemic shock and an increase is usually noted as volume is replaced.

An arterial catheter can be placed via any of several sites, including the radial, axillary, femoral, and brachial arteries. Most clinicians favor the radial artery because it is superficial and easily accessible. However, this artery may be difficult to cannulate in a hypotensive patient. The femoral artery is a large vessel that affords access even in patients with hypotension or vasoconstriction. The axillary and brachial arteries are infrequently used and should be avoided in the anticoagulated patient.

Insertion of the arterial catheter should be performed by clinicians experienced in the procedure. The insertion technique has been described in detail elsewhere (2,3). Complications associated with use of the arterial line include arterial thrombosis, embolization, hematoma formation, catheter-related infection, necrosis of overlying skin at the radial site, and retroperitoneal hemorrhage associated with femoral line insertion.

Pulmonary Artery Catheter

Since Swan et al (4) originally described the use of diagnostic heart catheterization, our experience with and knowledge gained from the pulmonary artery catheter (PAC) have substantially increased. This catheter has become an integral part of the management of critically ill patients suffering from oliguria, pulmonary edema, cardiac disease, sepsis, or shock, and those requiring vasoactive drugs and mechanical ventilation with high-pressure support. The hemodynamic parameters obtained with the Swan-Ganz catheter provide more accurate information than clinical signs and assist in selecting the optimal course of treatment. However, a criticism of invasive hemodynamic monitoring has been the lack of a randomized prospective trial demonstrating improved survival of critically ill patients through use of the PAC (5).

Often, accurate estimations regarding hemodynamic status can be made based on clinical information, but certain patients present a confusing clinical picture. Common indications for invasive monitoring in the obstetric patient are listed in Table 9.1. The PAC should be employed only when it is anticipated that management of the patient's condition will be altered by the hemodynamic information obtained. Relative contraindications include anticoagulation, recent thrombolytic therapy, and a hypercoagulable condition.

Table 9.1 *Indications for invasive monitoring in obstetrics*

I. Complications of preeclampsia
    A. Oliguria (< 30 mL/hr) unresponsive to fluid
       challenges that total 1000–1500 mL
    B. Hypertension unresponsive to initial agents and
       requiring vasoactive agents such as sodium
       nitroprusside
II. Hypovolemic shock unresponsive to fluid
    resuscitation
III. Septic shock requiring volume resuscitation or
    vasopressors
IV. Congestive heart failure or pulmonary edema not
    responsive to initial therapy
V. Respiratory compromise or adult respiratory distress
    syndrome requiring intubation
VI. Intrapartum or intraoperative management of
    A. Class III or IV heart disease
    B. Pulmonary hypertension

The information derived from this catheter must be carefully interpreted in the context of the normal values for pregnancy. Clark et al (6) demonstrated that gravid women have significantly increased cardiac output and heart rate, while systemic and pulmonary vascular resistance, colloid oncotic pressure (COP), and COP–pulmonary capillary wedge pressure (PCWP) gradient are decreased when compared to the nonpregnant state. No change was noted in MAP, PCWP, and left ventricular stroke work index (see Table 1.7).

The typical PAC is a triple-lumen, 7Fr polyvinyl catheter introduced into the central circulation via cannulation of the subclavian, internal jugular, or femoral vein and "floated" into the pulmonary artery. The catheter has multiple ports that allow direct measurement of heart rate, central venous pressure, pulmonary artery systolic and diastolic pressures, PCWP, cardiac output, and percent venous saturation. The data generated from the catheter can be used to calculate additional hemodynamic parameters that aid in determining the physiologic state of the patient. Since body surface areas have never been established for pregnancy, converting hemodynamic parameters to their respective "index" (e.g., cardiac index) remains controversial in the care of the obstetric patient.

It is crucial to correctly interpret and understand the hemodynamic information obtained from the PAC. PCWP is often the most clinically useful parameter, providing the patient has a normal mitral valve. The "wedge pressure" is obtained by inflating the balloon at the catheter tip that lies in the pulmonary artery. The wedge pressure reflects left atrial pressure and correlates with the degree of pulmonary congestion (Table 9.2). The pulmonary artery diastolic pressure is closely related to the mean PCWP and measures right atrial pressure (preload). Central venous pressure also reflects preload, and will be elevated in the presence of left ventricular dysfunction or overload. However, the central venous pressure and PCWP do not correlate in patients with severe preeclampsia, myocardial infarction, or mitral stenosis.

Table 9.2 *Correlation between pulmonary capillary wedge pressure and pulmonary congestion in the presence of a normal colloid osmotic pressure*

Pulmonary capillary wedge pressure	Pulmonary congestion
18–25 mm Hg	Mild-moderate
25–30 mm Hg	Moderate-severe
> 30 mm Hg	Pulmonary edema

Thus, in this group of patients the central venous pressure reading will not accurately reflect left-sided heart pressures, and placement of a PAC should be considered when a patient with any of these disease processes requires central monitoring.

The risks associated with insertion of the PAC include pneumothorax, ventricular arrhythmia, and catheter knotting. Infection, sepsis, pulmonary artery thrombosis, embolus or rupture, and pulmonary infarction are complications that can occur while the catheter is in place. It must be emphasized that a clinician experienced in the placement of the PAC attend this procedure. A complete description of the insertion technique is beyond the scope of this chapter and can be found elsewhere (7,8).

■ AMNIOTIC FLUID EMBOLISM

Amniotic fluid embolism (AFE) is an uncommon event, occurring most frequently during the intrapartum period. This syndrome may be the result of embolization of abnormal amniotic fluid into the maternal circulation, and it has been postulated that leukotrienes contribute to the maternal response (9). The overall mortality rate has been reported to be as high as 80% (10,11), with 50% of patients dying in the first hour after the onset of symptoms.

AFE has been described as a biphasic process characterized by a maternal hemodynamic response involving left-sided heart failure, pulmonary vascular injury, and a consumptive coagulopathy. The initial phase is one of hypoxia, systemic hypotension, pulmonary hypertension, and left ventricular injury. Although pulmonary artery spasm and secondary cor pulmonale have been suggested in the pathophysiology of AFE, left ventricular failure is the only hemodynamic aberration consistently documented in human subjects (12–14). It is possible that the pulmonary vascular changes occur very early in the course of the syndrome and simply have not been clinically documented owing to their transient nature. The second phase of AFE consists of left ventricular failure, a consumptive coagulopathy, and subsequently adult respiratory distress syndrome.

Patients with AFE classically present with acute respiratory insufficiency and systemic hypotension, followed rapidly by cardiorespiratory arrest. The diagnosis is based on this clinical presentation and exclusion of other causes of cardiopulmonary failure such as septic shock, aspiration pneumonia, acute myocardial infarction, pulmonary embolus, anesthetic toxicity, and placental abruption. No single laboratory or clinical finding is diagnostic of AFE. Although the presence of fetal squamous cells in the maternal pulmonary artery has been suggested as diagnostic of the syndrome, fetal cells and debris have been detected in patients undergoing pulmonary artery catheterization for indications other than AFE (15–17).

Treatment of this condition is aimed at oxygenation, maintenance of cardiac output and blood pressure, and correction of the coagulopathy. To prevent maternal central nervous system damage, ventilation with high-concentration oxygen is essential in the setting of profound hypoxia. An unconscious patient should be intubated and mechanically ventilated with 100% oxygen, and cardiopulmonary resuscitation (CPR) initiated when indicated. The initial treatment of hypotension includes rapid administration of crystalloid intravenous fluids. A dopamine infusion can be started when hypotension persists despite aggressive fluid resuscitation. Once the patient's blood pressure is stabilized, intravenous fluid administration should be decreased to a maintenance rate to minimize the risk of pulmonary edema. Pulmonary artery catheterization may be very useful in guiding further therapeutic interventions. In the presence of a coagulopathy, fresh frozen plasma, packed red blood cells, and platelets will be required to treat the bleeding diathesis. The patient's coagulation profile (prothrombin time, activated partial thromboplastin time, fibrinogen level, and platelet count) should be used to determine the need for individual components.

When a fetus is of a viable gestational age, the fetal heart rate must be carefully monitored for signs of compromise. Conversely, fetal distress has been reported to be the presenting sign in a patient with AFE (18). The decision regarding operative intervention must be individualized with consideration given to the maternal condition, the effects of resuscitative efforts, and the fetus' gestational age.

■ PERIMORTEM CESAREAN SECTION

Perimortem cesarean section affords the clinician an empiric approach to a viable fetus when immediate maternal survival is uncertain. This situation may arise in an already critically ill gravida or in an acute setting such as trauma, anesthetic catastrophe, massive embolism, or a cerebrovascular accident. It is important to emphasize that this procedure should not be undertaken in anticipation of maternal cardiac arrest but only in the event of actual cardiovascular collapse. The iatrogenic insult of an operative procedure can actually worsen a patient's condition and therefore worsen both the maternal and fetal outcome.

The issues of perimortem cesarean section focus on maternal as well as fetal physiologic considerations. Successful CPR depends on maintaining cardiac output by chest compressions, oxygenation, and medication administration as indicated (Table 9.3). Even under optimal conditions, CPR generates only 30% of the normal cardiac output. In the gravid patient, vena caval obstruction with supine positioning further reduces venous return to the heart and thus diminishes cardiac output. Unfortunately, left lateral tilt of the patient will only further reduce the effectiveness of the chest compressions. Anecdotal reports suggested more successful outcomes when the uterus is emptied (19,20). An additional consideration is that cesarean section is associated with significant blood loss, and this may further compromise the maternal condition unless volume replacement is initiated.

Table 9.3 *Medications used in cardiopulmonary resuscitation*

Drug	Dosage	Indication
Atropine	0.5–1.0 mg IV	Bradycardia
		Asystole
Epinephrine 1: 10,000	0.5–1.0 mg IV	Asystole
		Ventricular fibrillation
		Electromechanical dissociation
Lidocaine	1 mg/kg IVP	Ventricular fibrillation
		Sustained ventricular tachycardia
		Ventricular ectopy
Bretylium	5 mg/kg IVP	Ventricular fibrillation
		Ventricular ectopy
Procainamide	20 mg/min	Ventricular ectopy
		Sustained ventricular tachycardia

IVP = intravenous push

Fetal considerations include the fact that survival appears to depend on the timing of the cesarean delivery. Clinical and laboratory experience suggests that optimal fetal outcome is achieved when total asphyxia is minimized and delivery is accomplished within 4 to 6 minutes of cardiopulmonary arrest (21,22). If a patient undergoes successful CPR and the fetus has not yet been delivered, in utero resuscitation is likely and the fetus can be closely monitored for signs of recovery.

Although available data are based primarily on retrospective reviews and do not document whether such actions improve maternal or fetal survival, a reasonable approach to perimortem cesarean section includes the following:

1. Attempts at delivery of the fetus should be strongly considered within 4 minutes of the maternal cardiopulmonary arrest.
2. CPR should be continued throughout the procedure if there is the possibility of maternal survival.
3. Sterile conditions are unnecessary and valuable time should not be lost in preparing the operative field.
4. Given the reports of fetal survival beyond the 4- to 6-minute time limit, a fetus of viable gestational age with signs of life should be delivered without regard to the time since maternal cardiopulmonary arrest.

■ REFERENCES

1. Deckardt R, Fembacher PM, Schneider KTM, et al. Maternal arterial oxygen saturation during labor and delivery: pain-dependent alterations and effects in the newborn. Obstet Gynecol 1987;70:21.
2. Santos AC, Petrikovsky BM, Kaplan GP. Neurologic and muscular diseases. In: Dataa S, ed. Anesthetic and obstetric management of high-risk pregnancy. St. Louis: Mosby Year Book, 1991:147.
3. Amin DK, Shah PK, Swan HJC. The Swan-Ganz catheter: tips on interpreting results. J Crit Illness 1986;1:40–48.
4. Swan HJC, Ganz W, Forrester J, Marcus H, Diamond G, Chonette D. Catheterization of the heart in man with use of a flow-directed balloon-tipped catheter. N Engl J Med 1970;283:447–451.

5. Robin ED. The cult of the Swan-Ganz catheter. Overuse and abuse of pulmonary flow catheters. Ann Intern Med 1985;103:445–449.

6. Clark SL, Cotton DB, Lee W, et al. Central hemodynamic assessment of normal term pregnancy. Am J Obstet Gynecol 1989;161:1439–1442.

7. Clark SL. The pulmonary artery catheter: insertion technique and complications. In: Clark SL, ed. Critical care obstetrics. 2nd ed. Cambridge, MA: Blackwell Scientific Publications, 1991:62–69.

8. Amin DK, Shah PK, Swan HJC. The Swan-Ganz catheter: insertion technique. Practical pointers to minimize risk and maximize results. J Crit Illness 1986;1:38–45.

9. Azegami M, Mori N. Amniotic fluid embolism and leukotrienes. Am J Obstet Gynecol 1986;155:1119–24.

10. Courtney LD. Amniotic fluid embolism. Obstet Gynecol Surv 1974;29:169.

11. Morgan M. Amniotic fluid embolism. Anesthesia 1979;34:29.

12. Clark SL, Cotton DB, Gonik B, et al. Central hemodynamic alterations in amniotic fluid embolism. Am J Obstet Gynecol 1988;158:1124–1126.

13. Clark SL, Montz FJ, Phelan JP. Hemodynamic alterations associated with amniotic fluid embolism: a reappraisal. Am J Obstet Gynecol 1985;151:617–621.

14. Girard P, Mal H, Laine JF, et al. Left heart failure in amniotic fluid embolism. Anesthesiology 1986;64:262.

15. Clark SL, Pavlova A, Horenstein J, et al. Squamous cells in the maternal pulmonary circulation. Am J Obstet Gynecol 1986;154:104–106.

16. Lee W, Ginsburg KA, Cotton DB, et al. Squamous and trophoblastic cells in the maternal pulmonary circulation identified by invasive hemodynamic monitoring during the peripartum period. Am J Obstet Gynecol 1986;155:999.

17. Plauche WC. Amniotic fluid embolism. Am J Obstet Gynecol 1983;147:982.

18. Barrows JJ. A documented case of amniotic fluid embolism presenting as acute fetal distress. Am J Obstet Gynecol 1982;143:599.

19. DePace NL, Betesh SS, Kotter MN. ''Postmortem'' cesarean section with recovery of both mother and offspring. JAMA 1982;248:971.

20. Marx GF. Cardiopulmonary resuscitation of late-pregnant women. Anesthesiology 1982;56:156.

21. Katz VL, Dotters DJ, Droegemueller W. Perimortem cesarean delivery. Obstet Gynecol 1986;68:571.

22. Windle WF. Brain damage at birth. JAMA 1968;206:1967.

■ BACTERIAL INFECTIONS

Neisseria gonorrhoeae

Neisseria gonorrhoeae is a gram-negative diplococcus commonly found in the urogenital tract. Pregnant patients may harbor this bacteria asymptomatically within the endocervical canal for extended periods of time. This organism has also been associated with infection throughout the urogenital tract, rectum, and pharynx, and may on occasion present as disseminated infection. Gonorrhea is sexually transmitted, with a reported incidence in pregnancy ranging from 0.5 to 7.0% (1). Risk factors for infection include low socioeconomic status, nonwhite race, adolescence, and multiple sexual partners (2). Of increasing concern is the identification of penicillin-resistant strains of *N. gonorrhoeae*. Nearly 2% of gonorrhea infections in the United States are due to plasmid-mediated penicillinase-producing gonorrhea. In addition, several strains of chromosomally mediated resistant gonorrhea with documented resistance to multiple antimicrobial agents have been identified (3).

The diagnosis of gonococcal infection is usually made by isolating the organism on selective media such as Thayer-Martin medium. The recent development of antigen-specific rapid testing using an enzyme-linked immunosorbent assay and DNA probe technology may shorten the time required for diagnosis (4). Gram's stain can be used to make a presumptive diagnosis of gonorrhea, although other gram-negative diplococci are occasionally found as normal vaginal flora.

Increasing evidence has implicated gonorrhea as a causative agent in multiple pregnancy complications including premature rupture of membranes, preterm delivery, chorioamnionitis, postpartum endometritis, and neonatal sepsis (1). Gonococcal ophthalmia is a well-recognized infectious disease complication of the neonate caused by vertical transmission of this organism at the time of delivery. In an at-risk population, routine antenatal screening and treatment of gonorrhea are recommended. However, reinfection can occur, and follow-up testing at admission to the labor and delivery suite is recommended. Patients presenting in labor without prenatal care represent a particularly high-risk population for infection and therefore should be routinely cultured. Listed in Table 10.1 are recommendations for the treatment of uncomplicated anogenital gonorrhea during pregnancy. In patients with suspected or previously untreated infection, appropriate therapy should be initiated at admission. Because concurrent infection with *Chlamydia* species is common, culture and treatment for this pathogen should be included (see below). Testing for other sexually transmitted diseases, including syphilis and human immunodeficiency virus (HIV) infection, should also be performed.

Neonates with gonococcal ophthalmia should be iso-

Table 10.1 *Treatment of* Neisseria gonorrhoeae *during pregnancy**

Antibiotic	Dose	Comments
Ceftriaxone	250 mg IM	
Cefotaxime	400 mg PO	
Spectinomycin	2 gm IM	For penicillin-allergic patients
Amoxicillin and probenecid	3 gm PO 1 gm PO	Penicillinase-resistant gonorrhea

*Erythromycin (500 mg four times daily for 7 days) should be concurrently administered to treat presumed *Chlamydia* infection. Tetracycline and quinolones are contraindicated during pregnancy.

lated until after the initiation of therapy. Ceftriaxone (25–50 mg/kg/day) should be administered to the neonate as a single parenteral dose for 7 days. The neonate's eyes should be irrigated with saline or buffered ophthalmic solution. Topical ophthalmic antibiotic preparations are of no additional benefit when appropriate systemic antibiotics are given (5). However, these preparations are commonly given after delivery to all neonates as a prophylactic measure.

Chlamydia trachomatis

Chlamydia trachomatis infection is the most common bacterial sexually transmitted disease in women (6). It is responsible for syndromes involving the pulmonary, enteric, ocular, and genitourinary systems. The incidence of chlamydial infection in pregnancy ranges from 2 to 37% (7). This infection is more prevalent in high-risk groups such as those with low socioeconomic status, unmarried status, late prenatal care, multiple sexual partners, mucopurulent discharge, concurrent sexually transmitted diseases, or asymptomatic bacteriuria and those younger than 20 years.

Chlamydial infections in the urogenital tract exhibit a wide range of signs and symptoms. Cervicitis can result in a friable, edematous, inflamed cervix, cervical tenderness, and a mucopurulent discharge. Chlamydia infection may result in a urethral syndrome consisting of pyuria and dysuria. The infection may also follow an indolent, subclinical course and be asymptomatic in up to 50% of patients (8). Thus, in an at-risk population, routine antenatal screening is recommended.

The effects of chlamydial infection on pregnancy outcome remain unclear (9). Some studies suggested a link between infection with this pathogen and preterm delivery, preterm rupture of membranes, increased perinatal mortality, and postpartum endometritis (9). The results of these studies are controversial, however, and current evidence suggests that recent infection (documented by IgM positivity) probably conveys the greatest risk for these complications (10,11). Neonatal complications from the vertical transmission of chlamydia can result in either conjunctivitis or pneumonitis. The pulmonary complications develop during the first 3 months of life in up to 10% of infants born to mothers with active infection (12).

The "gold standard" for the diagnosis of chlamydial infection is culture in mammalian cell lines, most commonly McCoy cells. This process is time-consuming and requires proper collection and transport of the clinical specimen. A culture has 100% specificity and 90 to 95% sensitivity and results are available within 3 to 7 days. Nonculture techniques are now available to assist in rapid diagnosis of chlamydial infection, including direct fluorescent antibody staining, enzyme immunoassay, DNA probes, and polymerase chain reactions.

The intrapartum treatment for chlamydial infection should be liberally undertaken, particularly for patients with documented infection, known exposure to a partner with chlamydia, culture-proved gonorrhea, or physical findings consistent with infection. Several treatment options are available during pregnancy. Erythromycin (500 mg four times a day for 7–10 days) is a commonly employed therapy. Amoxicillin or clindamycin may be used in patients experiencing intolerance to erythromycin (13). A single dose of azithromycin (1 gm) has been used with good efficacy (14). Therapy for the partner is important, to diminish the possibility of reinfection. Neonates with known exposure to chlamydia are treated with erythromycin syrup after delivery; all newborns are routinely given ophthalmic prophylaxis.

Group B Streptococci

Group B streptococci (GBS) are well recognized as a leading cause of both maternal and perinatal infectious morbidity and mortality. In the parturient, GBS are associated with urinary tract infection, chorioamnionitis, and postpartum endometritis. More commonly, they can be asymptomatically identified as a component of the lower genital tract and rectal flora. Approximately 5 to 40% of pregnant women are carriers of GBS (15), and 40 to 70% of neonates born to colonized mothers will themselves be colonized (16). One to 2% of these colonized infants will subsequently develop invasive GBS disease in the form of early-onset sepsis (17,18). Given that most cases of early-onset GBS sepsis are acquired in utero, 70 to 80% of these neonates will have positive blood cultures at birth (19). Risk factors for GBS sepsis in the newborn are listed in Table 10.2 (20). Although multiple gestation is recognized as a risk factor, this may simply represent a confounding variable. Late-onset GBS infection presents outside the first week of life and typically presents with meningitis or failure to thrive. The attack rate for late-onset GBS is 0.5 to 1.0 case per 1000 live births.

The following approaches have been attempted to reduce the incidence of early-onset neonatal GBS sepsis:

- Postnatal chemoprophylaxis
- Antepartum identification and treatment of carriers
- Maternal immunization
- Antepartum identification and intrapartum chemoprophylaxis
- Intrapartum identification and chemoprophylaxis

None of the above-listed approaches will completely eradicate this disease process (21,22). Although the first option is simple to carry out, its efficacy is questioned. In addition, problems with penicillin-resistant pathogens in the nursery have been identified due to the broad use of this agent. There are no data to support the antepartum treatment of maternal GBS colonization in the otherwise asymptomatic patient (except as related to asymptomatic bacteriuria). This second option is therefore not recommended by most authorities. Maternal immunization, the third option, holds some promise

Table 10.2 *Risk factors for group B streptococcal (GBS) neonatal sepsis*

Premature labor

Preterm rupture of membranes

Prolonged rupture of membranes (>18 hr)

Intrapartum fever

Previous neonate with GBS sepsis

Heavy maternal GBS colonization

Absence of type-specific maternal antibody

Multiple gestation

owing to the recognized association between a deficiency in maternal antibody levels and risk for neonatal sepsis. Unfortunately, this approach may be limited by the fact that transplacental passage of protective antibodies is reduced prior to 32 weeks' gestation.

Intrapartum chemoprophylaxis appears to be the most promising method to reduce the incidence of early-onset disease. Selection of appropriate candidates for this approach remains controversial. Awaiting standard culture results from samples taken at admission to the labor unit is impractical in most instances. Therefore, many clinicians rely on antepartum culture results as a marker for intrapartum maternal colonization status. Recently, a variety of rapid diagnostic tests were marketed in an attempt to provide timely information regarding GBS positivity. Unfortunately, most of these new techniques have a limited sensitivity, especially with lightly colonized patients (23). Given the above-mentioned issues, a number of official agencies including the American College of Obstetricians and Gynecologists, the American Academy of Pediatrics, and the Centers for Disease Control have suggested management options based on various permutations of established risk factors and culture positivity.

The following are reasonable, but not absolute, recommendations for the prevention of neonatal GBS sepsis:

1. Screen for GBS colonization between 26 to 28 weeks by culturing the lower vaginal/anorectal regions using a methodology that maximizes recovery of the organism. Communication systems should be in place to reliably transmit this laboratory information to the labor unit.
2. Administer GBS *intrapartum* chemoprophylaxis to gravidas who are known to be GBS positive and have at least one recognized risk factor (see Table 10.2).
3. For women presenting to the labor unit with unknown GBS status, give intrapartum chemoprophylaxis if risk factors are identified. Cultures should be obtained, and subsequent management based on the outcome of these cultures if delivery of the baby has not occurred.
4. Antibiotic choices include intravenous penicillin G (5 million units every 6 hours) or ampicillin (2 gm every 6 hours) until delivery. In penicillin-allergic patients, either intravenous clindamycin (900 mg every 8 hours) or erythromycin (500 mg every 6 hours) can be substituted.

Amnionitis

Amnionitis is an infection involving the intrauterine con
tents prior to delivery, with an incidence ranging from
0.5 to 10.5% (24–26). It is defined as an acute, bacteria
mediated disease process, though other causative agent
such viruses and mycoplasmas have also been impli
cated. Two conditions frequently confused with the clin
ically overt presentation of intrapartum amnionitis are
incipient amnionitis (microbiologic evidence of bacteria
within the amniotic contents in an asymptomatic patient
and histologic chorioamnionitis (microscopic evidence o
inflammatory infiltrates within the placental mem
branes). These latter two conditions have distinctly dif
ferent maternal and neonatal concerns and outcomes
and therefore are not addressed in this section.

Amnionitis is usually an ascending infection, involv
ing aerobic and anaerobic, gram-positive and -negative
bacteria common to the lower female genital tract
Thirty-five to 70% of women diagnosed with amnioniti
have at least 10^2 colony-forming units (CFU)/mL iden
tified within the amniotic cavity (27). *Escherichia coli* and
GBS are frequently seen with amnionitis, especially
when bacteremia is present. The presence of organism
within the amniotic cavity does not always correlate
with clinical disease, and 8% of patients without overt
signs of infection have at least 10^2 CFU/mL (27)
Amnionitis has less frequently been the result of hema
togenous, transplacental spread. *Listeria monocytogenes*
group A streptococci, and *Campylobacter* species are
examples of infectious pathogens transmitted by thi
route.

Ascending infection usually follows spontaneous or artificial rupture of the fetal membranes, although infection has been reported with intact membranes. Risk factors include multiple digital examinations, prolonged membrane rupture, use of internal pressure catheters, prolonged labor, and the presence of higher concentrations of virulent organisms in the vaginal flora (e.g., associated bacterial vaginosis). These factors appear additive in causing amnionitis (24). Invasive procedures for diagnosis and therapy during pregnancy also place the patient at an increased risk for amnionitis. This complication results from direct inoculation of the amniotic cavity with local flora, and occurs with 0.1% of amniocenteses, 0.7% of percutaneous fetal umbilical blood samplings, and following 1 to 2% of cervical cerclages (24).

The primary feature of amnionitis is fever, although authorities differ on how this should be defined (i.e., a temperature > 37.8° versus 38.0°C). Additional nonspecific criteria include fetal and maternal tachycardia, foul-smelling discharge, uterine tenderness, and maternal leukocytosis. These clinical findings may be so variable that the presence of fever during labor alone usually allows for the presumptive diagnosis of amnionitis. Other obvious sources of infection, such as the upper respiratory and urinary tracts, should be excluded.

Certain laboratory data support the diagnosis of amnionitis. Amniotic fluid obtained transabdominally or through an intrauterine pressure catheter is the most useful specimen. Gram's stain of the amniotic fluid should be performed along with aerobic and anaerobic bacterial cultures. These microbiologic data are helpful in directing the empiric choice of antibiotics and guiding postpartum therapy, respectively. Under circumstance where the diagnosis of amnionitis is uncertain, a variety of adjunctive tests have been used in an attempt to support the diagnosis. These include measuring amniotic fluid glucose levels, leukocyte esterase activity, and cytokines, and determining an amniotic fluid white blood cell count. Gas-liquid chromatography has been used to identify organic acids within the amniotic fluid, which are by-products of bacterial activity. Although these adjunctive laboratory studies are of scientific interest, their generalized use in the clinical setting awaits further supportive documentation and commercialization.

Amnionitis is associated with an increase in maternal morbidity and mortality. It is the most common cause of septic shock in pregnancy. Prolonged and dysfunctional labor is frequently seen with amnionitis, along with an increased incidence of cesarean section for arrest disorders and fetal distress. Neonatal morbidity (specifically respiratory distress syndrome, intraventricular hemorrhage, and sepsis) is increased in association with amnionitis. Perinatal mortality is increased due to neonatal sepsis and prematurity, with a strong inverse relationship between gestational age and the consequences of amnionitis.

The specific goals in treating amnionitis are: 1) identification of the specific pathogen(s) responsible for amnionitis, 2) empiric antimicrobial therapy, 3) initiation or augmentation of delivery, and 4) close monitoring of mother and fetus for evidence of further compromise or distress. Amnionitis is likely to be a polymicrobial process and broad-spectrum antibiotic coverage should be promptly initiated. A typical regimen includes ampicillin (1–2 gm given intravenously every 6 hours) combined with an aminoglycoside (e.g., gentamicin, 100-mg intravenous load, then 80 mg every 8 hours). Subsequent dosing for the aminoglycosides should be adjusted based on serum peak and trough levels obtained after the third dose. Vancomycin (1 gm given intravenously every 12 hours) can be substituted for ampicillin in patients allergic to penicillin. Because patients undergoing cesarean delivery have a high failure rate when specific anaerobic coverage is not included, the addition of intravenous clindamycin (900 mg every 8 hours) or metronidazole (500 mg every 6 hours) is usually recommended. A number of advanced-generation antimicrobials have now been demonstrated to have efficacy as monotherapy for amnionitis. The clinician should feel comfortable utilizing these agents provided they are cost-effective and the institution can adequately screen for the development of resistant organisms. These agents should be safe for use in pregnancy and cross the placenta effectively. When combination therapy is used, a first-generation cephalosporin can be substituted for ampicillin in the patient with a history of mild penicillin allergy. Patients with a more significant history of penicillin allergy should be given vancomycin (1 gm intravenously every 12 hours) as a substitute.

Antibiotics should not be withheld until delivery, as studies clearly have shown benefit for both the patient and the neonate when the antibiotics are given promptly on diagnosis (28,29). Cesarean delivery is reserved for standard maternal and fetal indications. Antibiotics are typically continued following cesarean delivery until the patient is afebrile for longer than 24 hours. An even more liberal approach of discontinuing antibiotics immediately following vaginal delivery has been adopted by some institutions, owing to the lack of scientific proof for improved efficacy with extended use. Most would agree that prolonged antibiotic therapy is not necessary following discharge provided the patient demonstrates a prompt response to initial interventions.

The Sepsis Syndrome

Infection along with thromboembolic events, hypertensive disease, and hemorrhage account for approximately 70% of all maternal deaths (30). Although sepsis occurs infrequently in the obstetric patient, the clinician should be aware of the presenting signs and symptoms to prevent progression of this infectious complication. The pregnant or recently delivered parturient has the advantage of youthful resilience and immunocompetence. Conversely, physiologic alterations of pregnancy may mask early recognition of the septic patient and delay definitive treatment. Likewise, in the undelivered gravida, both mother and fetus must be given balanced consideration when instituting a management plan.

Sepsis is defined as a constellation of systemic physiologic and immunologic responses to infection (Table 10.3) (31,32). *Shock* is the inability of the body to maintain adequate cellular perfusion due to the above-cited host compensatory mechanisms. The infectious focus in the pregnant patient is most commonly chorioamnionitis, an abscess, pyelonephritis, peritonitis (i.e., appendicitis), or cellulitis. Prognosis for recovery from septic shock is correlated with the early identification

Table 10.3 *Definition of the sepsis syndrome**

Fever

Hypothermia

Tachypnea

Tachycardia

Impaired organ system function or perfusion

    Altered mentation

    Hypoxemia

    Elevated plasma lactate

    Oliguria

*Modified from Balk RA, Bone RC. The septic syndrome: definition and clinical implications. Crit Care Clin 1989;5:1–8.

and treatment of both the shock event and the inciting organism(s).

Clinically, septic shock can be divided into three distinct clinical phases: 1) early or warm shock, 2) late or cold shock, and 3) secondary or irreversible shock (33). These phases represent early physiologic responses to sepsis, overcompensation by the host's defense mechanisms, and finally end-organ dysfunction, respectively. Extreme of temperature is usually the earliest clinical sign in early shock. Shaking chills and tachycardia, along with nonspecific symptoms such as malaise, nausea, diarrhea, and agitation, are also encountered. Dyspnea and tachypnea are worrisome presenting signs because they may signal impending respiratory compromise and early-onset adult respiratory distress syndrome (ARDS). Initial hemodynamic changes consist of an increasing cardiac output along with a decrease in systemic vas-

cular resistance. Laboratory studies may show a leuko
penia or leukocytosis, mild thrombocytopenia, elevated
glucose concentration, and a mild respiratory alkalosis
on arterial blood gas analysis.

Reflex vasoconstriction results in transient improve
ment in cardiac output, but at the expense of hypoper
fusion and impaired oxygen delivery to the extremities
and central organs. Clinically, the patient may now be
cold, cyanotic, and oliguric, and have significant mental
status alteration. Further deterioration leads to multiple
organ system failures, including ARDS, renal failure, and
disseminated intravascular coagulopathy. Laboratory
changes reflect progressive coagulation derangements;
serum electrolyte measurements reveal an anion gap
as bicarbonate decreases and lactate levels rise, and
reduced renal function is signaled by rising serum cre
atinine and blood urea nitrogen levels. The later phases
of shock are associated with myocardial depression, fall
ing cardiac output, low systemic vascular resistance, and
widespread terminal vasodilation.

Management of septic shock centers around: 1)
maintaining optimal intravascular volume, cardiac out
put, blood oxygen-carrying capacity, and pulmonary gas
exchange while 2) identifying the source of the infection
and instituting appropriate medical or surgical therapy,
or both. The initial management of septic shock should
focus first on stabilizing the maternal condition, as
efforts to intervene on behalf of the fetus may have cat
astrophic results for both mother and baby. Fetal decom
pensation is closely related to the maternal condition and
its effect on uteroplacental perfusion. An exception to
this approach is when the fetal compartment is the septic

focus, which mandates prompt uterine evacuation while instituting stabilizing measures.

Therapeutic interventions should be employed to reverse the physiologic aberrations seen in septic shock. Oxygen administration at 10 L/min by face mask should be initiated and monitored with pulse oximetry. Circulating volume is replaced aggressively with crystalloid solutions. This replacement may be considerable due to extravasation of fluids associated with increased capillary permeability. One to 2 liters of normal saline or lactated Ringer's solution should be rapidly administered, and invasive hemodynamic monitoring instituted to guide further volume support. Fluids should be given with the goal of maintaining the pulmonary capillary wedge pressure (PCWP) at 10 to 15 mm Hg and optimizing left ventricular preload. Cardiac output, oxygen saturation, and systemic vascular resistance are additional invasive hemodynamic parameters that may assist in fluid management and guide additional therapeutic interventions.

Patients whose hemodynamic parameters do not improve after initial fluid resuscitation will need exogenous catecholamine or sympathomimetic support. Dopamine is the first-line vasoactive agent used by most clinicians, and has dose-related catecholamine-receptor selectivity (34,35). At a low dose (0.5–5.0 μg/kg/min), its primary action on dopaminergic receptors in the splanchnic, renal, and cerebral systems results in vasodilatation. As the dose is increased (5–10 μg/kg/min), beta-adrenergic effects predominate with a positive inotropic cardiac effect and minimal peripheral vasoconstriction. At high doses (> 10–15 μg/kg/min), the dominant alpha-receptor effects cause widespread peripheral vasoconstriction. The higher doses of dopamine are unfavorable in the treatment of shock because systemic perfusion is diminished and afterload and cardiac work are increased secondary to the alpha effect.

Dobutamine and norepinephrine are additional sympathomimetic agents that can be used in the treatment of septic shock. The beta-1- and beta-2-adrenergic effects of dobutamine provide both inotropic support and peripheral vasodilation. This may be an appropriate choice for the patient with low cardiac output as dobutamine improves output without increasing cardiac work or oxygen demand. Norepinephrine, in contrast, has predominantly alpha-adrenergic activity that affects peripheral vasoconstriction.

ARDS is a noncardiogenic form of pulmonary edema commonly encountered in sepsis. The patient demonstrates progressive hypoxemia, decreased pulmonary compliance, normal PCWP, and characteristic diffuse pulmonary infiltrates on chest radiographs (32,34). Respiratory failure with ARDS requires supportive measures aimed at maintaining ventilation and oxygenation. Intubation and mechanical ventilation are required when noninvasive respiratory support is unsuccessful. Ventilation with high-fractional inspiratory concentrations of oxygen are initially given, but the oxygen concentration should be decreased to nontoxic levels (< 50%) as soon as possible. Positive end-expiratory pressure is also frequently needed to maintain adequate oxygenation.

Equally important are identification and treatment of the septic source. A thorough search for the infectious etiology is essential to guide the antibiotic therapy and identify sites that require surgical drainage or debridement. Other studies, such as amniocentesis, ultrasound, computed tomography, and magnetic resonance imaging, may be indicated in an effort to locate the source of infection. Broad-spectrum aerobic and anaerobic parenteral antimicrobial coverage should be promptly instituted after appropriate cultures are obtained (33,35,36). A commonly used regimen includes a penicillin (penicillin G, 5 million units every 6 hours), an aminoglycoside (gentamicin, 100-mg load, then 80 mg every 8 hours), and anaerobic coverage with either clindamycin (900 mg every 8 hours) or metronidazole (500 mg every 6 hours). The aminoglycoside therapy should be carefully monitored in the septic patient with compromised renal function. Alternatively, aztreonam (2 gm given intravenously every 6–8 hours) may be substituted; this agent has excellent gram-negative coverage without significant renal toxicity.

When the uterus is the infectious source, delivery should be effected after initial stabilization of the patient. The mode of delivery depends on gestational age and the fetal condition. Vaginal delivery is the preferred route and can be accomplished in most cases. In the critically ill parturient remote from delivery, timely intervention with cesarean delivery may benefit both mother and baby. Meticulous surgical technique must be employed, including careful hemostasis, copious irrigation, and consideration for secondary wound closure. If a suboptimal response to antibiotic therapy is noted in the postpartum period, evaluation for abscess formation, secondary infection, and septic pelvic thrombophlebitis should be undertaken.

■ ANTIBIOTIC PROPHYLAXIS

General Principles

The intrapartum use of prophylactic antibiotics is intended to attenuate the risk of infection by reducing bacterial colonization or seeding at the time of delivery. The general principles regarding prophylaxis are well established (37,38) and support the need for adequate tissue concentrations at the time of contamination using an agent with appropriate antimicrobial coverage. Short-term antibiotic prophylaxis is usually adequate. Clinicians should be aware of periodic survey results regarding resistance patterns in their patient population. The cost-effectiveness of antibiotic prophylaxis is not necessarily based on the cost of the antimicrobial agent but rather on its benefit in reducing maternal morbidity, reflected as less need for therapeutic antibiotics and shortened hospital stays.

Cesarean Delivery

Antibiotic prophylaxis in the noninfected patient undergoing cesarean delivery has been shown to reduce postoperative febrile morbidity and endometritis. The benefit in decreasing wound infection or postoperative urinary tract infection is less well established. Although controversial, most authorities recognize specific risk factors for postoperative infectious morbidity, including labor, membrane rupture, multiple pelvic examinations, and internal pressure transducer monitoring (39). Obesity, anemia, and underlying medical conditions are less-specific risk factors. The timing of antibiotic administration is not as critical for cesarean delivery compared to other operative procedures. Efficacy has been demonstrated when the prophylactic agent is given preoperatively, at cord clamping, or immediately following surgery. Monotherapy using a broad-spectrum penicillin or cephalosporin-type agent is typically recommended (40). Single-dose prophylaxis is usually adequate (41). Patients with strong, immediate hypersensitivity to penicillin present a management dilemma. Either a combination of clindamycin (900 mg) and gentamicin (1.5 mg/kg), or metronidazole alone (500–750 mg) has been recommended empirically as alternative prophylaxis (42). Prophylaxis failure may be due to an already established incipient infection at the time of surgery, as opposed to inappropriate antibiotic selection or timing of administration (43).

Subacute Bacterial Endocarditis

The incidence of heart disease in women of reproductive age approximates 1%, and 5 to 10% of women have valvular lesions (44,45). With a decrease in rheumatic heart disease, most acquired lesions result from an increase in intravenous drug abuse. In patients at risk, subacute bacterial endocarditis can occur during the delivery process and involves the seeding of anatomically abnormal cardiac structures with bacteria endogenous to the procedure site. This transient bacteremia may only last 15 to 20 minutes. The American Heart Association recommendations can be found in Chapter 2 and Table 2.4.

Manual Removal of the Placenta and Uterine Curettage

There are no standard recommendations regarding the need for antibiotic prophylaxis during manual removal of the placenta or postpartum uterine curettage. It seems reasonable to presume that these procedures may place the patient at increased risk for postpartum endometritis. If antibiotics are used for prophylaxis, a regimen similar to that recommended for cesarean section could be utilized.

■ VIRAL INFECTIONS

Herpes Simplex Virus

Genital herpes simplex virus (HSV) infection is a sexually transmitted disease caused by the HSV type 1 or 2. The incidence of genital herpes in the general population is 1 to 2%. HSV has been documented in the genitourinary system of 0.4 to 7.4% of patients during pregnancy (46). Primary or recurrent herpes infection can be a source of maternal morbidity but more importantly can result in severe neonatal morbidity and mortality. Herpes infections can be classified as primary infection (defined by the absence of maternal antibodies), first-episode nonprimary (antibodies present), and recurrent episode (47). First-episode nonprimary and recurrent HSV outbreaks can occur throughout pregnancy and are not associated with an increase in abortion or low-birthweight infants (48). Conversely, an increased risk of adverse pregnancy outcome with primary disease has been reported (49).

Primary infection in the gravida may result in severe localized pain, high fever, urinary retention, mental status changes, seizures, and liver abnormalities. Hospitalization may be required for patients with severe systemic symptomatology. Under these circumstances, acyclovir, an antiviral agent that inhibits HSV DNA polymerase, has been used primarily in the interest of maternal well-being (50,51). Acyclovir is given either intravenously for 5 to 7 days (5 mg/kg of body weight, over 45–60 minutes, every 8 hours) or orally for 7 to 10 days (200 mg five times daily). Patients who have a primary outbreak during the third trimester should be followed with serial cultures until a negative culture is documented, in order to offer subsequent vaginal delivery (49). *Recurrent* HSV rarely leads to significant maternal morbidity, and therefore pharmacologic intervention is relatively contraindicated during pregnancy. There appears to be no advantage to serial culturing of the asymptomatic gravida with a history of genital HSV infection as this is a poor predictor of viral shedding at the onset of labor (52).

Prevention of perinatal transmission to the neonate is the major concern during the intrapartum period. The incidence for delivering HSV-infected neonates from parturients with viral shedding at the time of labor is from less than 4% for those with recurrent or asymptomatic disease to 50% for those with primary HSV (53). It is estimated that 1.4% of patients with a history of HSV infection will be shedding virus at the time of delivery (53). Patients with a history of HSV infection should be identified prenatally and carefully examined at presentation in labor. If no lesions are present and no prodromal symptoms are elicited (burning, pruritis, paresthesia, and pain), vaginal delivery can be offered. A recurrence site-specific and cervical culture may be obtained from the patient on presentation or directly from the newborn after delivery, to identify neonates exposed to women with asymptomatic shedding. In patients with active lesions or prodromal symptoms, cesarean delivery is indicated to reduce the risk of neonatal herpes infection. Cesarean delivery should be performed within 4 to 6 hours of membrane rupture, although the neonate may still benefit from operative intervention despite a longer delay (52).

Recently, a great deal of interest has focused on the prophylactic use of acyclovir to reduce the risk of HSV recurrence at the time of delivery. Proponents argue that the drug carries no identifiable risk to the fetus (based on ongoing registry data) (54) and reduces clinical recurrences in the nonpregnant patient when used in this fashion. Of interest, one study using prophylactic acyclovir in the general population did not show a decrease in the incidence of asymptomatic viral shedding (55). Investigations currently underway are examining the prophylactic use of acyclovir late in pregnancy and its effect on viral shedding, cesarean delivery rate, and neonatal infection.

Hepatitis Viruses

For a complete discussion on hepatitis, the reader is referred to Chapter 4.

Human Immunodeficiency Virus

HIV infection is a retroviral disease of significant importance. Women with HIV infection comprise the fastest growing group of infected individuals in the United States (56). It is estimated that there are 250,000 cases of diagnosed acquired immunodeficiency syndrome (AIDS or symptomatic HIV infection) and perhaps a million antibody-positive asymptomatic people in the United States. Women comprise 10 to 12% of the HIV-positive group in America, with most cases epidemiologically associated with illicit drug use. The incidence of HIV antibody positivity in the general obstetric population is estimated to be 1 in 1000, while in high-risk populations this increases to 1.0 to 1.5% (56).

The course of HIV infection involves four stages (56). Following initial infection, the patient has a mononucle-osis-like illness as the virus is actively replicating and invading all of the body's tissues, especially the lymphatic system. This is followed by an asymptomatic latent phase (as long as 10 years) in which the patient is antibody positive and viral replication continues at a low rate. The third stage involves mild to moderate symptoms along with the surfacing of opportunistic diseases. The final stage is marked by overt immunodeficiency, cachexia, and life-threatening infection. Life expectancy is 5 years or less once the patient becomes symptomatic (57). Although controversial, being a woman, or pregnancy itself, does not appear to alter the outcome of HIV infection if all other variables are comparable.

The recommendation to perform routine prenatal screening for HIV antibody status has gained acceptance as specific benefits continue to be recognized for the mother and fetus. Barbacci et al (58) showed that screening limited to patients in high-risk groups will identify only 57% of HIV-positive women. In one study, four independent risk factors for HIV infection were: 1) use of crack cocaine, 2) more than two sexual partners, 3) sexual intercourse with a high-risk partner, and 4) testing positive for syphilis (59). These risk factors are often difficult to elucidate from patients for a variety of social and logistical reasons. Prenatal screening must always be performed under conditions of confidentiality with adequate pretest and posttest counseling available.

During pregnancy, the HIV-infected gravidas should be screened for sexually transmitted diseases, tested for associated infections such as tuberculosis, and receive appropriate vaccinations. CD4 cell counts should be serially monitored as a marker for disease progression. Most importantly, even asymptomatic patients with CD4 cell counts higher than 200 per cubic millimeter should be offered treatment with zidovudine (100 mg five times daily). Therapy begun between 14 and 34 weeks' gestation and continued in labor recently was associated with a reduction in the rate of vertical transmission from 25.5 to 8.3% (60). Intrapartum zidovudine therapy is started with the onset of labor (2-mg/kg intravenous loading dose) and a constant infusion (1 mg/kg/hr) is continued throughout labor (60). Because this new therapeutic recommendation is based on data from a single study, additional investigations should be conducted to confirm this beneficial effect of zidovudine prophylaxis.

Care must be taken to avoid intrapartum procedures such as scalp electrode placement, scalp pH sampling, and vacuum extraction that may empirically increase the risk of fetal infection (61). Though some believe that mode of delivery may influence the rate of vertical transmission (62), prospective studies showed similar rates of transmission for cesarean and vaginal births (63). Therefore, at the present, cesarean delivery should only be undertaken for obstetric indications.

Information gathered from large multicenter studies

shows an approximate risk of 0.3% for health care workers who are inadvertently pricked with a contaminated needle from an HIV-positive patient (64). Although this apparently low occurrence rate is reassuring, it is important to maintain ongoing educational programs for hospital staff related to universal precautions to further limit this exposure risk.

Varicella-Zoster Virus

Varicella-zoster virus is a DNA virus in the herpesvirus family that causes chickenpox. Although varicella is an uncommon adult infection, approximately 5% of women in the reproductive age group are seronegative (65). Varicella is a highly contagious disease with an incubation period of 10 to 20 days. The disorder is self-limiting in children, but significant morbidity, including high fever, skin lesions, encephalitis, and pneumonia, can occur in adults. Pregnancy itself does not predispose a nonimmune patient to varicella infection, but may result in a more morbid disease course.

The most serious complication of adult varicella infection is pneumonia, which has been reported in up to 50% of patients (66,67). Respiratory symptoms can surface as early as 2 days after the appearance of the skin lesions. Patients should be counseled to seek physician care if they develop pleuritic chest pain, dyspnea, hemoptysis, or cyanosis. Health care providers need to be aware that hospitalization and full respiratory support may be necessary for these patients. Acyclovir and adenosine arabinoside (ARA-A) are two pharmacologic agents that can be used to treat this pulmonary complication (68). Acyclovir acts as a DNA polymerase inhibitor, and is the drug of choice in this setting. It is administered intravenously at 5 to 10 mg/kg over 1 hour and repeated every 8 hours for up to 7 days. ARA-A (10 mg/kg/day for 5 days) is also a DNA polymerase inhibitor but does not have the same selective antiviral effect as acyclovir. Central nervous system side effects have been associated with its use, and therefore ARA-A is reserved for patients with an inadequate response to acyclovir.

Fetal considerations involve exposure to the varicella-zoster virus around the time of delivery. If delivery takes place 5 days before or after the onset of maternal infection, the reported risk of life-threatening neonatal varicella-zoster virus infection is 17%, with a subsequent mortality rate of 31% (69). This is thought to be due to the lack of maternal varicella antibody production within this window of time. If delivery does occur during this critical time, 1.25 mL of varicella-zoster immune globulin (VZIG) should be administered to the neonate immediately following delivery. Empiric neonatal acyclovir therapy may also be appropriate.

Patients who present near term with a recent exposure to varicella and no history of previous infection present a management dilemma. McGregor et al (70) reported that most women (71%) will have demonstrable antibodies, and 90% of those with indeterminate histories were immune. Intramuscular VZIG administration (625 units in multiple injection sites) within 96 hours of maternal exposure may ameliorate the maternal effects of the disease while protecting the fetus during the viremia. Testing for the presence of maternal varicella antibody should be undertaken if the status is unknown.

Seropositivity will exclude the group of patients not needing expensive VZIG administration.

Human Papillomavirus

Human papillomavirus (HPV) infection may be the most common sexually transmitted disease in women (71). HPV is a DNA virus, infection with which can present clinically as condylomata acuminata or flat condylomata. Subclinical infection is the more common presentation and may be detected by routine Papanicolaou smear or with specific DNA probes. HPV has been detected in up to 30% of sexually active females (72), and its prevalence is likely to be similar in the pregnant population (71). Antepartum care of clinically significant HPV infection may include ablative measures with trichloroacetic acid (TCA), cryotherapy, or laser therapy depending on the location and extent of the lesions. The clinical benefit of interventional therapy during pregnancy, to either the mother or the fetus, has yet to be definitively elucidated. Evaluation of an abnormal Papanicolaou smear with appropriate studies and follow-up care should be included as part of the patient's antepartum care.

There are two basic intrapartum concerns in the patient with HPV infection. In patients with large, bulky vaginal or vulvar lesions, obstruction to passage of the fetus through the birth canal can occur, albeit infrequently. Episiotomy or perineal body lacerations involving extensive lesions can be extremely difficult to repair and may be associated with significant hemorrhage. For these reasons, cesarean delivery may be indicated in the interest of maternal well-being. The second concern relates to the neonate and focuses on the risk of developing juvenile laryngeal papillomatosis (JLP), the most common benign childhood tumor of the larynx. Whether perinatal exposure to HPV results in development of these multiple papillary growths on the larynx remains controversial (73). Clinical onset of JLP is before age 5 in 50 to 75% of patients (74). This condition may lead to significant morbidity and possibly death from upper airway obstruction. Conservative estimates place the risk of the neonate acquiring JLP from an infected mother at 1 in 400 to 1 in 1500 (74), although this is the subject of intense debate. While cesarean delivery has been suggested by some as a preventative approach to JLP, one case of JLP has occurred following cesarean delivery with intact membranes (75). At this time, cesarean delivery is not routinely advocated to prevent JLP in the neonate born to mothers with HPV infection, although patients should be counseled regarding this potential complication. Following delivery, it should be anticipated that maternal HPV genital lesions will regress.

■ ACKNOWLEDGEMENT

This chapter was written with the assistance of Dr. Michael McNamara, Clinical Instructor, Department of Obstetrics and Gynecology, Wayne State University School of Medicine, Detroit, MI.

■ REFERENCES

1. Sweet RL, Gibbs RS. Sexually transmitted diseases. In: Infectious diseases of the female genital tract. 2nd ed. Baltimore: Williams & Wilkins, 1990:109–43.
2. Dallabetta G, Hook EW III. Gonococcal infections. Infect Dis Clin North Am 1987;1:25–54.

3. Centers for Disease Control. Antibiotic-resistant strains of *Neisseria gonorrhoeae*. Policy guidelines for detection, management and control. MMWR 1987;36(S):1–18.

4. Osen JV, Michael MF. Experience with modified solid phase enzyme immunoassay for detection of gonorrhea in prostitutes. Sex Transm Dis 1986;13:1–4.

5. 1993 Sexually transmitted diseases treatment guidelines. MMWR 1993;42(RR-14):62.

6. Livengood CH. Chlamydial infections. In: Gleicher, N, ed. Principles and practice of medical therapy in pregnancy. 2nd ed. Norwalk, CT: Appleton & Lange, 1992:613–26.

7. Sweet RL, Gibbs RS. Chlamydial infections. In: Infectious diseases of the female genital tract. 2nd ed. Baltimore, MD: Williams & Wilkins, 1990:45–74.

8. Sexually transmitted diseases. In: Cunningham FG, MacDonald PC, Gant NF, Leveno KJ, Gilstrap LC, eds. Williams obstetrics. 19th ed. Norwalk, CT: Appleton & Lange, 1993:1304–5.

9. Gibbs RS, Romero R, Hillier SL, Eschenbach DA, Sweet RL. A review of premature birth and subclinical disease. Am J Obstet Gynecol 1992;166:1515–28.

10. Sweet RS, Landers CV, Walker C, Schachter J. *Chlamydia trachomatis* infection and pregnancy outcome. Am J Obstet Gynecol 1987;156:824–33.

11. Berman SM, Harrison HR, Boyce WT, Haffner WJJ, Lewis M, Arthur JB. Low birth weight, prematurity, and post partum endometritis. JAMA 1987;257:1189–94.

12. McGregor JA, French JI. *Chlamydia trachomatis* infection in pregnancy. Am J Obstet Gynecol 1991;164:1782–89.

13. Centers for Disease Control. Sexually transmitted diseases treatment guidelines, 1993. MMWR 1993;42(RR-12):1–39.

14. Bush MR, Rosa C. Azithromycin and erythromycin in the treatment of cervical chlamydial infection during pregnancy. Obstet Gynecol 1994;84:61–63.

15. Group B streptococcal infections in pregnancy. ACOG Technical Bulletin No. 170. American College of Obstetricians and Gynecologists, Washington, DC, July 1992.

16. Katz VL. Management of group B streptococcal disease in pregnancy. Clin Obstet Gynecol 1993;36:832–42.

17. Greenspoon JS, Wilcox JG, Kirschbaum TH. Group B streptococcus: the effectiveness of screening and chemoprophylaxis. Obstet Gynecol Surv 1991;46:499–508.

18. Boyer KM, Gotoff SP. Antimicrobial prophylaxis of neonatal group B streptococcal sepsis. Clin Perinatol 1988;15:831–50.

19. Christensen KK, Christensen P, Lindberg A, et al. Mothers of infants with neonatal group B streptococcal septicemia are poor responders to bacterial carbohydrate antigens. Int Arch Allergy Appl Immunol 1982;67:7–12.

20. Dinsmoor MJ. Group B streptococcus. In: Zuspan FP, Quilligan EJ, eds. Current therapy in obstetrics and gynecology. Philadelphia: WB Saunders Company, 1994:221–223.

21. Ohlsson A, Myhr TL. Intrapartum chemoprophylaxis of perinatal group B streptococcal infections: a critical review of randomized controlled trials. Am J Obstet Gynecol 1994;170:910–17.

22. Department of Health and Human Services/Centers for Disease Control and Prevention. Prevention of group B streptococcal diseases: a public health perspective. Fed Reg 1994;240:64764–73.

23. Yancey MK, Armer T, Clark P, Duff P. Assessment of rapid identification tests for genital carriage of group B streptococci. Obstet Gynecol 1992;80:1038–47.

24. Gonik B. Amnionitis. In: Zuspan FP, Quilligan EJ, eds. Current therapy in obstetrics and gynecology. Philadelphia: WB Saunders Company, 1994:208–10.

25. Soper DE, Mayhall CG, Dalton HP. Risk factors for

intraamniotic infection: a prospective epidemiologic study. Am J Obstet Gynecol 1989;161:562–8.

26. Newton ER. Chorioamnionitis and intraamniotic infection. Clin Obstet Gynecol 1993;36:795–808.

27. Gibbs RS, Duff P. Progress in pathogenesis and management of clinical intraamniotic infection. Am J Obstet Gynecol 1991;164:1317–26.

28. Sperling RS, Ramamurthy RS, Gibbs RS. A comparison of intrapartum versus immediate postpartum treatment of intra-amniotic infection. Obstet Gynecol 1987;70:861–65.

29. Gibbs RS, Dinsmoor MJ, Newton ER, Ramamurthy RS. A randomized trial of intrapartum versus immediate postpartum treatment of women with intra-amniotic infection. Obstet Gynecol 1988;72:823–28.

30. Atrash HK, Koonin LM, Lawson HW, Franks AL, Smith JC. Maternal mortality in the United States, 1979–1986. Obstet Gynecol 1990;76:1055–60.

31. Fein AM, Duvivier R. Sepsis in pregnancy. Clin Chest Med 1992;13:709–22.

32. Balk RA, Bone RC. The septic syndrome: definition and clinical implications. Crit Care Clin 1989;5:1–8.

33. Gonik B. Septic shock in obstetrics. Clin Perinatol 1986;13:741–54.

34. Rackow EC, Astiz ME. Pathophysiology and treatment of septic shock. JAMA 1991;266:548–54.

35. Boyd JL, Stanford GC, Chernow B. The pharmacotherapy of septic shock. Crit Care Clin 1989;5:133–50.

36. Lee W, Clark SL, Cotton DB, et al. Septic shock during pregnancy. Am J Obstet Gynecol 1988;159:410–16.

37. Duff P. Prophylactic antibiotics for cesarean delivery. A simple cost effective strategy for prevention of postoperative morbidity. Am J Obstet Gynecol 1987;157:794–98.

38. Ledger WJ. Antimicrobial agents. In: Ledger WJ, ed. Infec-

tion in the female. Philadelphia: Lea & Febiger, 1986: 113–20.

39. Enkin M, Enkin E, Chalmers I, Hemminki E. Prophylactic antibiotics in association with cesarean section. In: Chalmers I, Enkin M, Keirse MJ, eds. Effective care in pregnancy and childbirth. Oxford: Oxford University Press, 1989:1246–69.

40. Faro S, Marteus MG, Hammill HA, Riddle G, Tortolero G. Antibiotic prophylaxis: is there a difference? Am J Obstet Gynecol 1990;162:900–9.

41. Gonik B, McGregor J. Comparison of short vs. long half-life single dose prophylactic antibiotics for cesarean section. Infect Dis Obstet Gynecol 1994;2:3–9.

42. Duff P. Antibiotic selection for infections in obstetric patients. Semin Perinatol 1993;17:367–78.

43. Gonik B, Shannon RL, Shawer R, Costner M, Seibel M. Why patients fail antibiotic prophylaxis at cesarean delivery: histologic evidence for incipient infection. Obstet Gynecol 1990;79:179–84.

44. McCurdy CM, Nolan TE. Endocarditis review and update on prophylaxis in the obstetric and gynecologic patient. Female Patient 1993;18:20–28.

45. Henderson CE, Terrible S, Keefe D, Merkatz IR. Cardiac screening for pregnant intravenous drug abusers. Am J Perinatol 1989;6:397–99.

46. Nenrukar LS, Jensen LP, McCallum P, et al. Frequency of asymptomatic genital herpes in pregnant women at term. Obstet Gynecol Surv 1988;43:132–34.

47. Gibbs RS, Sweet RL. Maternal and fetal infections. In: Creasy RK, Resnik R, eds. Maternal fetal medicine: principles and practice. Philadelphia: WB Saunders Company, 1994:666.

48. Kulhanjian JA, Soroush V, Au DS, et al. Identification of women at unsuspected risk of primary infection with her-

pes simplex virus type 2 during pregnancy. N Engl J Med 1992;326:916–20.

49. Brown AZ, Vantuer LA, Benedetti J, et al. Effects on infants of a first episode of genital herpes in pregnancy. N Engl J Med 1987;317:1246–51.

50. Brown ZA, Baker DA. Acyclovir therapy during pregnancy. Obstet Gynecol 1989;73:526–531.

51. Corey L, Fyfe K, Benedetti J, et al. Intravenous acyclovir for the treatment of primary genital herpes. Ann Intern Med 1983;98:914–921.

52. Arvin AM, Hensleigh PA, Prober CG, et al. Failure of antepartum cultures to predict the infant's risk of exposure to herpes simplex virus at delivery. N Engl J Med 1986:315;796–98.

53. Trofatter KF Jr. Herpes simplex viruses. In: Gleicher N, ed. Principles and practice of medical therapy in pregnancy. 2nd ed. Norwalk, CT: Appleton & Lange, 1992:638–43.

54. Acyclovir in pregnancy registry, international surveillance. Epidemiology, and Economic Research Division, Burroughs Wellcome Company, 3030 Cornwallis Road, Research Triangle Park, NC 27709.

55. Strauss SE, Seidlin M, Takiff HE, et al. Effect of oral acyclovir treatment on symptomatic and asymptomatic virus shedding in recurrent genital herpes. Sex Transm Dis 1989;16:107–13.

56. Duff P. Human immunodeficiency virus infection in pregnancy. Semin Perinatol 1993;17:379–83.

57. Human immunodeficiency virus infections. ACOG Technical Bulletin No. 165. American College of Obstetricians and Gynecologists, Washington, DC, March 1992.

58. Barbacci M, Repke JT, Chaisson RE. Routine prenatal screening for HIV infection. Lancet 1991;337:709–11.

59. Ellerbrock TV, Lieb S, Harrington P, et al. Heterosexually transmitted human immunodeficiency infection among

women in a rural Florida community. N Engl J Med 1992; 327:1704–07.

60. Connor EM, Sperling RS, Gelber R, et al. Reduction of maternal-infant transmission of human immunodeficiency virus type 1 with zidovudine treatment. N Engl J Med 1994;331:1173–80.

61. Viscarello RR. Human immunodeficiency virus infection in obstetrics and gynecology. In: Pastorek JG, ed. Obstetric and gynecologic infectious disease. New York: Raven Press, 1994:579–607.

62. Paz I, Seidman DS, Mashiach S, Stevenson DK. Maternal transmission of human immunodeficiency virus-1. Obstet Gynecol Surv 1994;49:577–84.

63. European Collaborative Study. Risk factors for mother-to-child transmission of HIV-1. Lancet 1992;339:1007–12.

64. Jagger J, Hunt EH, Brand-Elnagger J, et al. Rates of needle-stick injury caused by various devices in a university hospital. N Engl J Med 1988;319:284–88.

65. Enders G. Varicella-zoster virus in pregnancy. Prog Med Virol 1984;29:166–96.

66. Smego RA Jr, Asperilla MO. Use of acyclovir for varicella pneumonia during pregnancy. Obstet Gynecol 1991;78: 1112–16.

67. Eder SE, Apuzzio JJ, Weiss G. Varicella pneumonia during pregnancy: treatment of two cases with acyclovir. Am J Perinatol 1988;5:16–18.

68. Ramin SM, Gilstrap LC. Varicella zoster in pregnancy. In: Pastorek JG, ed. Obstetric and gynecologic infectious disease. New York: Raven Press, 1994:343–51.

69. Meyers JD. Congenital varicella in term infants: risks considered. J Infect Dis 1974;129:215–17.

70. McGregor JA, Mark S, Crawford GP, Levin MJ. Varicella zoster antibody testing in the care of pregnant women exposed to varicella. Am J Obstet Gynecol 1987;157:281–84.

71. Kemp EA, Hakeneworth AM, Laurent SL, Gravitt PE, Stoecker J. Human papillomavirus prevalence in pregnancy. Obstet Gynecol 1992;79:649–56.

72. Osborne NG, Adelson MD. Herpes simplex and human papillomavirus genital infections: controversy over obstetric management. Clin Obstet Gynecol 1990;33:801–11.

73. Hallden C, Majmudar B. The relationship between juvenile laryngeal papillomatosis and maternal condyloma acuminata. J Reprod Med 1986;31:804–7.

74. Kashima HK, Shah K. Recurrent respiratory papillomatosis: clinical overview and management principles. Obstet Gynecol Clin North Am 1987;14:581–88.

75. Shah K, Kashima H, Polk DF, et al. Rarity of cesarean delivery in cases of juvenile-onset respiratory papillomatosis. Obstet Gynecol 1986;68:795–99.

Index

▼   ▼   ▼   ▼   ▼